"I'll Never Have Sex with You Again!"

Tales from the Delivery Room

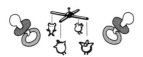

IRENE ZUTELL and LARRY BLEIDNER

A Fireside Book

Published by Simon & Schuster

New York   London   Toronto   Sydney   Singapore

FIRESIDE
Rockefeller Center
1230 Avenue of the Americas
New York, NY 10020

FIRESIDE and colophon are registered trademarks
of Simon & Schuster, Inc.
For information about special discounts for bulk purchases,
please contact Simon & Schuster Special Sales:
1-800-456-6798 or business@simonandschuster.com
Designed by Helene Berinsky
Manufactured in the United States of America
10 9 8 7 6 5 4 3 2 1
Library of Congress Cataloging-in-Publication Data is available.
ISBN 0-7432-1464-1

This book is dedicated to moms everywhere—especially our own.

To Magdalen and Catherine.

And to Olivia, our daughter,

whose arrival into the world was the inspiration for this book.

CONTENTS

INTRODUCTION

*E*ureka moments always strike at the oddest times. There I was, legs splayed by stirrups, privates exposed and a 6-pound, 13-ounce creature ramming its head at my cervix. A pain coursed through my body that made me pray for death. And then my husband and my obstetrician nearly came to blows.

I thought, Wouldn't this make a funny book?

Let me back up a bit: A few days before my due date, my doctor—the one I had interviewed for the job, the one I thought *understood* me and my unborn child—decided to mention that he'd be plying the Greek isles during my baby's birth. He walked me to the office of his partner, wished me luck and sailed off humming the theme from *The Love Boat.*

I was left facing Dr. Brock St. Claire, the substitute obstetrician, who seemed more like an actor playing a doctor than the real deal. But this was Hollywood, where even brain surgeons sneak out for auditions during lunch breaks. He shook my hand and stretched his face into a crescent-moon smile. His teeth were so white and polished they belonged behind glass, spread out on a swatch of black velvet. His skin was mahogany from too many sessions at an electric beach. His perfectly coiffed hair was just this side of a televangelist's.

This guy's going to deliver my baby? I panicked and then

squinted past his head, desperately searching for diplomas and various degrees. All I discovered were headshots of actresses and models. *Thanks, Brock, for catching my baby. You're the best,* one read. He caught me looking and raised his eyebrows. It was as if he were saying, Oh yeah, I've seen their vaginas.

Eventually I calmed down. St. Claire may not be the Norman Rockwell–doctor I'd imagined, but if a bunch of millionaire actresses trusted him with their labor, why shouldn't I? Besides, it was too late to search for someone else.

A few days later I was in the delivery room. St. Claire barreled in and announced, "We'll have this bambino out in a few minutes." Then he imparted some medical advice. "Just keep pushing like you're taking a shit. I like to tell my patients that this is the biggest shit of their lives."

As he laughed, St. Claire checked his reflection in the mirror that had been positioned by my legs. He smiled.

"Remember, push like you're really constipated, honey."

I squeezed my husband's hand and we took long, deep breaths together. Sweat dripped down my face as the contractions tore through me. I'd been pushing for the last two hours. I wanted more drugs. I wanted to call it quits. I wanted a doctor to slice me open and pull this creature out. I wanted to die.

Then St. Claire said: "So, if it's a boy, I'll circumcise him."

I held my breath, pushed and waited. I'd heard Larry's take on circumcision so many times now I had it memorized. Our original doctor knew the deal but apparently St. Claire hadn't checked the files. During the last nine months, Larry had debated this with everyone—friends, family, co-workers, waiters, mailmen, winos . . .

"No way."

Even though Larry and I didn't know our child's sex, he was convinced it was a boy. He'd been calling my swollen stomach "Johnny" for the last nine months. And he had made it clear from the moment the plus sign appeared on the EPT test that his son's foreskin would remain intact. Since Larry believed he knew more about penises than I did, he thought he should have the final say in this matter. Jeannine, my sister, had a solution. "Just have the baby circumcised and then blame it on the drugs." *Gee, I really don't remember anything.* . . .

Most people quickly abandon a debate with Larry on this subject. Believe me, it's not worth it. Larry's a master at verbal sparring. I suppose most decide, "Sure, let his kid be ruined for life. Why should I care?"

St. Claire's mouth hung open. His teeth glistened under the fluorescent light. "*No!!!!!!!!????* You can't be serious. Everyone gets their kid circumcised."

St. Claire was on one side of me. My husband on the other. They were like two matrons across a picket fence.

Larry gritted his teeth as he spoke. "I don't. Why mess with the manufacturer's original design?"

"Why? Because . . . because you don't want your son to be a freak. And you don't want your son giving women bladder infections because of all the smegma. He'll have too much smegma."

My baby hadn't even been born yet and already he was a sex machine!

"Smegma? Please." Larry ignored my contraction as he clenched his jaw. "Circumcision is no different from tattooing or body piercing. It's mutilation."

The nurse strapped an oxygen mask to my face while St. Claire swatted his hand through the air as if Larry's remarks were the dumbest things he'd ever heard. The nurse cleared her throat. "Doctor, this baby is ready to come out."

St. Claire thrust his palms out at the nurse to silence her. After all, there were more important issues at hand. "Well, I'd like to know who's going to clean the smegma."

The baby was ripping my bowels. I pushed. "It's almost there. We're at stage two," the nurse said. "Look, you can see its head."

The hairy top of my precious baby's head was showing and the doctor and my husband ignored it. Instead they glared at each other.

"Why stop at the foreskin? Why not lop off a couple of inches so his pants fit better?"

I pushed and pushed. I exhaled and inhaled. I visualized. I was on a raft—alone—in the ocean, floating peacefully. The cool water lapped at my legs. The sun massaged my face, my shoulders, my arms, my stomach . . .

St. Claire threw up his arms and guffawed. "You're circumcised, right? You know the trauma your child will go through when he sees that your penises are different?"

"You know, I was worried about that." Then Larry pretended to cup his penis as he spoke in a good ol' voice. "Lookie here, Junior, our Johnsons don't match."

St. Claire's eyes narrowed. "You laugh now. But what about the kids in the locker room? You think it will be easy for him if his penis is different from theirs? He'll be ridiculed. He'll have no friends. He'll come home from school begging you to cut his penis. What will you do then, huh? *Huh?*"

"I'll get him a box-cutter and a fifth of Jack Daniel's."

My ocean churned with turbulence. The raft capsized. I swallowed gallons and gallons of salt water. A shark bore through my stomach. I was dying! And they were talking about smegma. When this was over, I'd report St. Claire to the American Medical Association, or the Screen Actors Guild. I'd file for divorce. Better still, I'd kill them both.

"GET THIS BABY OUT OF ME," I barked at the doctor. I turned to my husband. "I'LL NEVER HAVE SEX WITH YOU AGAIN!!!!!!!!"

After I'd uttered this anthem for laboring moms, that eureka moment hit. I thought, This can't be an isolated incident of delivery-room hijinks. With pain at a maximum and adrenaline on overdrive, childbirth captures people at their most insane. Why not a book that takes a lighthearted look into this extraordinary event? After all, I couldn't be the only mom yelling, *"I'll never have sex with you AGAIN!"* Could I?

After my delivery, I recounted the story to friends. My suspicions were confirmed—many had hilarious anecdotes to share. There's the father who missed his son's delivery so he could change into a suit and tie. The mother-in-law who grabbed the forceps and demanded that the doctor get busy. The nurse who relentlessly pitched a horror movie to a mom giving birth. And the wife about to undergo a cesarean who believed her husband was plotting her murder. As one labor nurse explained, "Women in labor get downright weird." But let's not be sexist. As another said, "The biggest laughs I've had are always at the expense of men in the delivery room. They just get so nervous."

"Tell me about when I was born." As children, it's one of the first stories we request because we're the main character. It's the first chapter of our lives and we can't get enough of it. We listen for Mommy and Daddy to fill us in, begging them to repeat parts until we have it memorized. It's family lore. I'd heard the story of my arrival so many times I'd forgotten what a wonderful anecdote it was. As my mother recounted it for the book, I realized I knew it verbatim, even though I hadn't heard it in decades.

So why not share these stories with expectant moms? After all, no one deserves a laugh more than pregnant women. They've got mood swings, hemorrhoids and an additional twenty-plus pounds to lug around. Plus everyone—friends, relatives, strangers on the street—feels compelled to share birthing horror stories with them. Larry and I promise that in this book there will be no sad stories or scary moments. All these stories have happy endings.

Which brings us back to my story.

Suddenly they remembered I was there. My husband squeezed my hand. "Okay, breathe, honey," he said. Yeah, as if I hadn't been doing it on my own for the last thirty years! You're worthless, I thought. I should be squatting in a field of sunflowers without any husbands, doctors or other variety of men around—circumcised or not.

"It's almost out," the nurse yelled.

A head appeared, followed by the tiniest, pudgiest, most wrinkled hand I'd ever seen. "Looks like it's reaching for a credit card," St. Claire said.

It felt as if everything inside me was tumbling out.

"What is it? What is it?"

"You tell me," the doctor said to Larry as he yanked the baby into the room at 1:11 P.M. on September 30, 1999.

"It's a girl! It's a girl!"

Thank God. A girl! A girl with indoor plumbing. A girl who couldn't be a freak in the locker room! A girl! The doctor placed the slimy, bloody, wriggly little creature on my chest. I wrapped my arms around her naked body and Larry cut the umbilical cord. We stared at our baby and fell in love.

I had my little family; and Olivia Jeannine, her first story.

"I'll Never Have Sex with You Again!"

I Am *Not* Out of Control!

Ladies, there's one time in your life when you get a free pass for outrageous behavior, and this is it.

Here's how some moms let fly with thoughts, words and actions.

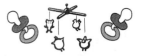

C'MON, ADMIT IT—
YOU REALLY ENJOYED THAT SHAVE

Jeannine Schwing is my (Irene's) sister, mom to Paul and Cate and one of the funniest people we know. Of course she'd have something to say about her delivery.

I'm terrified of hospitals. Even if I just drive past one, my heart races and I feel sick to my stomach. When I became pregnant, I blocked the hospital part from my mind and imagined the baby magically appearing.

That's probably the reason I didn't go into labor. My due date came and went. A week passed. A few more days. Four years later, I'd probably still be carrying this baby to avoid the hospital. However, the doctor decided it was time to induce.

I was extremely nervous. We arrived at the hospital at six thirty in the morning on March 18. They took us into labor and delivery.

They hooked me up to Pitocin to trigger labor. A few minutes later I felt a tightening, which was the start of contractions. Dave, my husband, was sitting near me watching *The Price Is Right*. Even today, when I hear that show's theme song or Bob Barker's voice, I feel like puking.

The doctor said I was dilating and asked if I wanted an epidural. I said yes. I wasn't in a ton of pain, but I was uncomfortable. My mother brags about having this very high threshold of pain. She's had teeth pulled without a drop of Novocain. I, however, need anesthesia when having my teeth cleaned. In the background, Bob Barker yelled for someone to "Come on down!" Behind Bob, some slinky model with a French manicure smiled and stroked a microwave like it was her lover's butt.

The doctor kept checking me. At 2 P.M., I was at nine centimeters, but the head wasn't coming down. He said by 4 P.M. I'd have the baby. But 4 P.M. came and went. He said, "Wait a little longer."

Suddenly the room was filled with beeping. *Beep-beep-beep-beep!* A nurse ran in. She looked at the fetal monitor, picked up a phone and told the doctor to come in right away.

Seconds later the doctor raced into the room. He looked at me. "We need to do a C-section right now." They pulled the gown off me. Then another nurse arrived and started shaving my pubic hair. She had the same nails as Bob Barker's model. I saw Dave watching the shaving. He looked like he was viewing a porno movie. He gave the nurse this big smile. I thought he was going to ask her to shave him, too.

I was paralyzed with fear. I thought I was going to die. Then the doctor hands me some paper to sign.

"You have to sign this," he said.

"Why?"

"In case you die."

I felt as if signing the papers would give the doctor permission to let me die. At first I refused. It was like signing my obituary, I thought. But Dave convinced me to sign. Maybe he had a life insurance policy out on me. I could see him in some cheesy

Vegas hotel room, lying on a heart-shaped, red velour bed. His face ecstatic as the same nurse shaved his pubes—all on my death benefit!

As they're prepping me for surgery, a nurse hands Dave scrubs.

Next thing, Dave's staring intently at my doctor. I realize he's trying to figure out how to wear the outfit. He starts getting dressed in his scrubs. He puts on his pants and shirt and checks himself in the mirror between my legs. My legs are actually shaking with fear, and my husband's completely oblivious. He spends what seems like hours adjusting the cap on his head. He's trying different angles. "How does the hat look?" he asks me. "Is this the same way Doctor H. wears it?"

I'm about to die and my husband is worried about how a hat looks. I don't even answer him. I just watch as he adjusts the mask over his mouth. I know he's enjoying this. He's pretending he's a doctor. In a muffled voice, he asks me how he looks again. I pretend I can't understand him. (I do that even when I'm not about to give birth.)

Everything worked out fine. Our son, Paul, was born at 6:52 that evening, weighing 7 pounds, 3 ounces. I'm still alive. Dave looked like an idiot in scrubs. And I still don't trust nurses. Especially ones with razors and French manicures.

ONE DAMN *RUDE* BABY!

After three kids, June Conklin of Ossining, New York,
thought she was a real expert when it came to childbirth.

I had the easiest childbirths ever. I was knocked out for the first one, so I barely knew I had the baby. The second one, I went into labor as I was getting my hair cut. I finished the trim at 4:30 P.M. and had my baby at four minutes after six that night. It slid right out of me. With the third one, I got a little cocky. I started getting contractions, but since my husband had just gotten home from work, I let him sleep. By the time we got to the hospital, the baby just popped out.

They say it gets easier with each child. With the fourth one, I figured I could practically squat in a field. Throughout my whole pregnancy I thought, This will be an easy one. My others were only two hours each, so why would this be any different? I'm very lucky, thank God. There are some people who are just made to have children and some who aren't. I, obviously, am born to breed and I'm proud of it.

I always thought my outlook helped a lot, too. You see, I have this philosophy about childbirth. It's all about what you make of it. If you're strong-minded and focused, you can just push the baby out—no problem. I also believe that you should never ever find out what you're having. The suspense helps the birthing. I believe that there's nothing like curiosity to help you push out that kid. I had it all figured out.

I began to suspect that I might not know as much as I thought I did. I'd been at the hospital for two hours with my fourth child and nothing had happened. At two in the morning, I should have had the baby already, but I was only two centimeters dilated. I kept saying, "When is this going to happen because this is getting ridiculous." I'm a very impatient person.

My doctor looked at me and says, "Well, everything's stopped."

I said, "What do you mean everything's stopped? It doesn't feel like everything's stopped. If everything's stopped, why am I in pain? Your machine must be broken. Get another machine."

As we're debating this back and forth, I'm listening to a woman in another room. She's screaming at the top of her lungs. I know this will sound sick, but I start smiling as this woman is screaming bloody murder. Misery loves company, I guess. Her shrieks are somehow comforting to me. It's nice to know that someone's in more pain than you. Ten minutes pass and the screams are like music to my ears. Then they just stop. I figure she must be vomiting or something. Maybe she died. I wait for the screams to begin again, but they don't.

A nurse comes into my room. I ask about the screamer down the hall. Is she dead? "No," the nurse says. "She had her baby." I ask her, "Was it her first one?" "Yes," the nurse tells me. "It's a beautiful baby girl."

Well, that's it. Suddenly, I'm pulling myself out of the bed and yelling, "THAT'S NOT FAIR! I WAS HERE BEFORE HER. I'M SUPPOSED TO HAVE MY BABY FIRST! THAT'S NOT FAIR. THIS IS MY FOURTH. IT SHOULD BE OUT ALREADY. I SHOULD HAVE BEEN THE ONE, NOT SOME FIRST-TIMER."

My mother's in the room and she starts crying hysterically. She thinks her daughter has completely lost it. My husband is looking at the monitor. He nudges me. "You're about to have a little contraction. It's no big deal."

No big deal? Well, that just sends me over the edge.

"WHO ARE YOU TELLING ME WHAT'S LITTLE AND WHAT ISN'T? YOU'RE JUST SITTING THERE, DOING NOTHING. WHAT DO YOU KNOW? YOU DON'T KNOW PAIN. YOU COULDN'T HANDLE THIS. THAT WAS NOT A LITTLE CONTRACTION. THAT WAS A *HUGE* CONTRAC-TION. THAT WAS OFF THE SCALE. WHO THE HELL DO YOU THINK YOU ARE?"

My doctor looks at my husband and says, "Why don't you leave for a little while. Get something to eat."

I'm getting these stabbing pains that I'd never had with my other children. I feel like my insides are being ripped apart. I'm screaming. I'm crying. And the doctor's telling me I'm not even ready to push. I was supposed to have this baby in an hour and it had been more than three hours! Like I said, I'm not a patient per-son. If I have an appointment, I'm always a half hour early. As far as I'm concerned, this baby is being rude. It should have been here already.

My husband comes back in the room with coffee and a muffin for himself. I'm in the worst pain of my life and he's stuffing his face with food like he's watching a football game or something.

I couldn't take it anymore. I jump out of the bed. I rip off my gown. I try to pull off all the cords that are attached to me. My mother's saying the rosary. My husband and the doctor are trying to hold me down. I scream at the top of my lungs: "I'M A PATIENT. I HAVE MY RIGHTS AND I WANT A C-SECTION RIGHT NOW. I'VE HAD ENOUGH OF THIS!"

Well, the last thing I had ever wanted was a C-section. I went through all my childbirths and not one stretch mark! Not one. Now, a C-section scar would be worse than any stretch mark, but I didn't care. The doctor looks at me and doesn't say a word.

"IF YOU'RE NOT GOING TO HELP ME, I WANT ANOTHER DOCTOR. I WANT TO GO TO ANOTHER HOSPITAL. I DON'T NEED THIS. I HAVE MY RIGHTS."

My husband's yelling at me to calm down. My mother's sobbing away. She's convinced I've lost my mind. She's praying. I'm trying to untangle myself from all the cords so I can get to a nice hospital where they'll give me a C-section without any hassles.

They give me some Demerol. Nothing happens. Actually, the pain gets worse.

I'm standing there yelling at my doctor. "CHECK THE EXPIRATION DATE ON THOSE. THEY'RE NOT WORKING. I FEEL EVERYTHING. WHAT KIND OF HOSPITAL IS THIS? YOU HAVE OLD USELESS DRUGS. THIS IS RIDICULOUS."

I'm going on and on about my rights when suddenly I feel this pressure. After three births, I know it's the head. I have to sit. I push twice and the baby's out. Just two big pushes and Lee-Ann popped out weighing 6 pounds, 4 ounces. She's born at 4:04 A.M. on August 1, 1994. Now that's more like it. That's what I'm used to.

I look around the room. My mother's mascara is pouring down her face. My husband looks like he might pass out. My doctor is pale. I'm beaming as I stare at my beautiful baby girl.

"That wasn't so bad," I say.

THE GERM BOAT

Jessica, a mom from Queens, New York, tells how a dream vacation in paradise turned into a nightmare cruise to hell.

$\mathcal{I}$'m a very suggestible person. If I watch a TV show with a hypnotist in it, I fall into a trance right in my living room. If I'm driving on the expressway and hear a police siren, I know I'm headed to jail. If I have a phone conversation with somebody who has a cold, by the time I hang up, my throat is sore. That's just the way I am. Not exactly a hypochondriac, but not all that far off, either.

When I first became pregnant, this germ thing of mine went into some kind of hyperdrive. I had two bodies to worry about, doubling my fun. When my husband, Mark, would come home from work, I'd make him wash his hands before he could touch anything. If anyone I knew had a cold, I'd avoid him or her until I was sure they were over it. Before the baby, I never cared about nonsmoking anything—in fact, I smoked through college and for a few years afterward. But with the baby, if someone lit a match on my block, I'd have a fit.

Now when I look back, I realize I wasn't so much fun to be around, and though he won't admit it, Mark started working later so he'd get to spend a little less time with *moi*. Mark is in sales, and all those extra hours he put in helped him win us a very nice vacation. It was a week-long eco-cruise around Central America, everything included. It was also a "use it or lose it" deal, so we had to go right away.

I had been to the Caribbean—you know, Bahamas, Puerto Rico, Virgin Islands—and loved it all. White beaches, palm trees, coconuts—what's not to like? Well, I really wasn't paying all that close attention to the "eco" part of the thing. So I agreed.

So we bought khakis, sun hats and number 30 sunscreen,

packed our bags and headed–by limo–for the airport. This was going to be great!

We flew to Costa Rica and had a nice night in a hotel. The next day, we were driven to the cruise ship. It looked okay, but it was a lot smaller than other cruise ships I'd seen; and the back of the boat looked weird. Our cabin was a little claustrophobic, but the crew couldn't have been nicer (or cuter–Ricky Martin must have cousins in Costa Rica).

The first night, they had a slide show to tell us about tomorrow's activities. We had a choice. We could take a guided hike through the rain forest or do some kayaking around the ship. Okay, since I was a little over four months, I figured paddling around in a kayak would be easier. Mark said, "Hey, you'll be bored with that in ten minutes–let's go see what's in the jungle."

When did they decide to call the jungle the rain forest? "Rain forest" sounds so nice. "Jungle" sounds so dangerous. I answered my own question, didn't I?

We had dinner, and the next morning we headed for adventure in the "rain jungle." That's when I found out why the back of the boat looked strange. I was expecting the ship to pull up to some big pier and we'd all walk down the gangplank and into a jungle lined with souvenir shops. No. We had to climb into rubber rafts, with little outboard motors, and then jump out when they hit the beach. It was like *Saving Private Ryan,* without the bullets. By the time we got halfway to the beach my clothes were soaked. Then, with the water landing, my feet were soaked, too. And it wasn't eighty and sunny. It was like fifty and heavily overcast.

If I could have hailed a cab right there to take us back to Queens, I would have–even if it meant selling the house to pay the fare. But I reminded myself to keep an open mind. Mark seemed to be enjoying himself. We started walking into the jungle.

Everything this guide stopped to show us could either make you really sick, or kill you. Spiders the size of squirrels. Bats. Bats hanging upside down, waiting for dark so they could swoop into your face. Then the guide waves to us like he's found Blackbeard's treasure or something. He shushes everyone and points at something under a tree. I forget what he called it, but it looked like a ten-pound rat with legs as long and thick as a pig's. And these people are smiling at it and snapping pictures like it's Elvis resurrected or something. I'm thinking, *What was I thinking?*

We hike a little farther and invade capuchin monkey territory. Again, I had figured there'd be one or two up in a tree a few miles away, but this was like being inside the monkey house at the zoo. They were all around us, and right over our heads, screeching and leaping. I started screeching as I raced back down the trail in the opposite direction. I'm thinking, I'm out of here. Eco-schmeko, this is not vacation, and God knows what diseases I am picking up from spiders and monkeys and giant rats. I walked back to the beach and made one of those guys take me back to the ship in the rubber raft.

At dinner, some woman who had spent the day kayaking sat at our table and asked me about the hike. I told her the monkeys were all I could stand. She looked at me and said, "They all have TB. And those bats? All bats carry rabies!" Rabies. Rhymes with babies. Jesus Christ!

The next day, I stayed on the boat. And the day after. And the day after. Finally, they announced they're pulling into some port. I'm thinking, Great—civilization! I can shop and see some concrete. But an hour before they docked, they canceled shore leave because of an outbreak of dengue fever in town. I asked a Ricky Martin how this fever, which could be fatal, was carried. By close personal contact or mosquito, I was told. I ran to the cabin and never left. Better cabin fever than dengue fever.

When I got home, I ran to my OB/GYN and told him everything. He calmed me down and said that if I'd gotten any kind of bug, I'd be showing symptoms by now. As soon as he said that, I started burning up. I made him take my temperature, but it was perfectly normal. I think he was laughing at me, but I didn't care.

So, for the next few months, I took my temperature daily, hardly left the house and prayed that neither my baby nor I had picked up any amoebas, microbes, spores or monkey-borne TB in the rain jungle.

Even when I went into labor, I couldn't stop thinking about dengue fever. Once the serious pushing started—and I pushed for two hours—I forgot all about it. Then, when my boy was in my arms, that was it! Heaven. John was born on March 3, 1995, weighing 7 pounds, 9 ounces. He was perfectly healthy.

Having John has calmed me down a lot. I don't worry about germs as much—with a kid, they're hard to avoid. Although I can guarantee you won't find either of us in any monkey house anytime soon!

I'LL TAKE MINE WITH PEPPERONI

B. J. Rack, a film producer (*T-2, Mimic, Beautiful*) from Los Angeles, could have used a stunt double for her daughter Sara's birth.

Our first child, Amy, had been a Lamaze adventure—no stress, low lights, only four and a half hours total—and transition was eleven minutes, very Zen. Of course, you always expect the next one to be the same. No way. Sara's debut was going to be the yin to Amy's yang.

It was October 7, 1983. We were living in the Hollywood Hills at that time. At about 2:30 A.M., I felt one lightning-bolt of a contraction. I pivoted upright, called my brother who lived a few blocks away and told him to come over to watch my youngest. Then I threw on a coat and woke my husband by screaming, "GET THE CAR!" I was certain that I was having the baby at any second.

We jumped in the car and flew to Cedars-Sinai. How fast was the baby coming? Well, I had a total of ten contractions before she was born. I was certain I wasn't going to make it to the hospital, and as we drove past major intersections, I starting thinking I'd name her after whichever boulevard she'd be born at. "Beverly" seemed pretty good. But when we hit Fairfax and Robertson, I abandoned that idea. Between those thoughts, I was screaming at my husband to pull over. "I'M HAVING THIS BABY NOW!" Finally, he took my word for it and pulled to the curb. But at that exact spot, I could see the hospital. Now I'm yelling, "DON'T STOP! GO!"

He pulls up in front of the hospital and I get out of the car, and he says, "I'm going to go park the car." So off he goes to park the car, and I feel like this baby is going to fall out of me.

I run into the reception area screaming, "I'M HAVING THE BABY! I'M HAVING THE BABY!" The receptionist very calmly says, "May I have your Social Security number?" I give her the number, and she starts to slowly type it into the computer. Then some guy comes over—an orderly or somebody, I never found out for sure—and starts wrapping that blood pressure–thing around my arm. I'm certain I'm about to drop this baby in a straight-back chair, and I spot a gurney. I feel like I need to be in a prone position and head for the gurney, which starts to rip the blood pressure sleeve from its mooring on the wall. This gets the orderly very, very nervous. He's saying, "No, ma'am, we have to take your blood pressure." He was being very nice about it, and I'm sure he assumed I was just another hysterical mother hours away from delivery.

I sit back down in the chair because now I feel I won't make it to the gurney. I realize I'm still wearing underpants, and all I can think is that I have to get them off me or the baby will suffocate. This poor guy is still trying to take my blood pressure when I dug my nails an inch into his arm and screamed in his face—"I'M HAVING THIS BABY NOW!" Well, I guess that did it. Suddenly this look of realization comes over his face and he says, "We better get you onto a gurney."

He helps me onto the gurney and says he's going to get a doctor. That's when I latch on to him again and say, "YOU'RE NOT LEAVING ME; YOU'RE HELPING ME HAVE THIS BABY!" Meanwhile, my husband is prowling the parking lot in search of the perfect parking space. And this orderly is pleading with me to let go of him so he can get a doctor. Even in my blind panic and excruciating pain, I negotiate a compromise and convince him to wheel me along as he looks for a doctor.

He finally wheels me into a room. I can feel that the baby's head is coming out, but I still have my panties on. The room is very dimly lit—no one can seem to find the light switch. They haven't yet located the doctor and in walks a nurse. The nurse helps me get my panties off and the baby starts coming faster. At that second the doctor walks in, followed by my husband, somebody hits the light switch, the baby shoots out of me and hydroplanes across the metal top of the gurney, right to the edge—and is stopped by the umbilical cord.

I look at the baby and she is an ashen blue color, which is not all that uncommon, but it convinces me she's somehow suffocated. I start screaming, "WHY IS SHE BLUE? WHY IS SHE BLUE!?!??!" Of course, the baby is screaming, too, and I just didn't realize that suffocated babies tend not to scream. Someone points that fact out to me and I begin to calm down a little bit.

The chaos begins to subside, the baby stops crying, the pain abates and my husband tells me the whole thing took maybe twenty minutes. I was never really quite checked into the hospital. I'm starting to feel better, and I turn to my husband and say, "Let's just go home." They weren't having any of that, so they wheel me into this recovery room and that's when a hunger that you wouldn't believe hits me. I ask for some food and they offer to get me some Jell-O and a fruit cup. That sounded about as satisfying as a glass of water and a stick of celery. So when the hospital people left the room, we ordered a pizza. I could see the nurses' station through the curtain and told the pizza guy to just bring it there. When it arrived, my husband swooped out, paid for it and brought it into the room. It was terrific. The best pizza I'd ever had.

And by the way, they never did get my blood pressure!

HEY, MOM, YOU GONNA KISS YOUR BABY WITH THAT MOUTH?

Bridget, a mom of two from a suburb of Baltimore, Maryland, was possessed by Andrew Dice Clay during her delivery.

$\mathcal{I}$ was at two centimeters for about eight hours, so everyone just assumed this was going to be a long, slow labor. The doctor went home for dinner. The nurses were tending to other patients. But suddenly everything felt very different. The contractions were tighter, stronger and closer. "This baby's coming," I said. My husband replied, "Oh no, honey. Don't worry about it, the doctor said you're only at two centimeters."

I was seeing red. How dare he tell me about *my* body! I commanded my husband to get the g.d. nurse. NOW! He took his own sweet time with it. When she finally checked me, she explained that I had gone from two to nine centimeters. I could give birth pretty soon.

Well, I was in pain and I wanted an epidural. From the moment I found out I was pregnant, I was all about modern medicine. None of this hero stuff for me. Drug me up. Make me numb. The problem? They said they couldn't find anyone to administer it. But I didn't believe it—I thought they wanted me to suffer. And I knew there was a time limit. If I didn't get the epidural soon, I'd never be able to have it.

I screamed, "I want my epidural now. I won't have the baby without it!"

The nurse had this thick Irish accent. "Relax. Calm down. Everything's all right." She kept saying this over and over and stroking my hair. "You're doing a lovely job. Relax, lovey." I couldn't take it anymore. She kept calling me honey, lovey, dear. I knew she was trying to stall the epidural, so I said, "Shut the fuck up! SHUT THE FUCK UP!"

Once I got the epidural, the pain disappeared, but I was mortified. I don't usually have a foul mouth. I felt horrible because she was the nicest nurse. I apologized and apologized. She said, "Oh, that's no big deal. I've been bitten, scratched and punched. Cursing is nothing."

2

They Like to Be Watched

For some women, giving birth is one of life's most private acts.

For others, it's a spectator sport. These moms prefer a crowd.

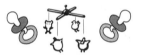

LIVE WITH REGIS

Catherine Jirak, a mom from the suburbs of New York City, tells how she became a TV star.

*M*y sister's friend had gotten us some tickets for a show called *LIVE with Regis & Kathie Lee.* This was 1988 and, believe it or not, I'd never heard of the show or this guy named Regis. I was about five weeks away from giving birth and I thought this would be a nice distraction.

My mom said, "You better not go into the city. You could have that baby any day."

I just laughed. Typical mom being dramatic. After all, I had more than a month until my due date.

So Alice, my sister, and I went to the show. It was okay. I don't remember too much about it. We were in the lobby getting ready to leave when I started to feel queasy.

"You know what, I don't feel right," I told Alice. "And I'm leaking."

I didn't know anything. It didn't even occur to me that I could be in labor. How could I? I'd only been to two Lamaze classes!

I tried to go into the bathroom, but there was a line of women about a mile long. Someone saw me and yelled, "Let her in. There's a pregnant woman here!" But this is New York and a bunch of people chimed in, "Yeah, so what. There are three other pregnant women on line and they're not looking for special treatment."

I walked into the men's room, which was filled with women. As I went inside, my water broke. It was gushing everywhere. Alice is a nurse, but she never had to deal with babies, and she was panicking. The first thought that ran through both of us was, Mom's going to kill us. She told us not to go. Then my sister starts yelling, "Has anyone here had a baby before?"

I'm in a stall for about twenty minutes as this water is just pouring out of me. Alice is outside on the phone trying to figure out what to do. To this day, I'm really not sure who she called. I don't think she knows, either.

As much as I wanted to, I realized I couldn't just stay in the men's room all day. I'm drenched, but I walk out and guess who's waiting there? Regis and the camera crew. I'm like, "Hi. This is just what I need." But they're rolling tape.

"I hear there's some excitement here," Regis said. I'm having seismic contractions and they're interviewing me. Regis asked me how I liked the show.

"It was okay."

He flipped. "Okay? What do you mean, okay?"

They followed me outside as we tried to hail a cab. I didn't want to call an ambulance because they take you to the closest hospital. We wanted a cab to drive us to our car that was parked on the Upper East Side. From there, I figured Alice could take me to my hospital in Westchester.

Finally, a cab stopped. Regis was still kibitzing as I was getting inside the cab. Then the cabdriver realized he was in the presence of none other than Regis Philbin and decided it was time for chitchat.

"Hey, Reege, remember me?" Then Regis and the cabdriver have a conversation for what seems like forever. My sister said, "Will you stop talking and go already! She's having a baby."

The cab took off and pretty soon we were in our own car. While Alice gunned the accelerator all the way down the Taconic State Parkway, I asked her questions. "What does it mean when your contractions are three minutes apart?" I mean, she did go to nursing school. But she keeps saying, "I don't know. I don't know. I know I read about it, but I forgot that chapter."

Conveniently, the baby waited until we arrived at the hospital. She was born a few hours later at four in the afternoon on October 19, 1988, weighing 6 pounds, 7 ounces. All night, the producers from the Regis & Kathie Lee show called for updates. Then at 8 A.M., Regis interviewed me over the phone. They showed the tape from the day before. A year later they had me on the show with baby Alison. So that was my few minutes of fame.

But when my sister and I tell the story, what makes us laugh the hardest has nothing to do with Regis or the show. We still can't believe how quickly we reverted to childhood and kept saying, "Oh my God, Mom is going to kill us."

OF COURSE IT WORKED.
HE MADE YOU VOMIT, DIDN'T HE?

Usually, one doesn't associate the occult with childbirth, but apparently in some exotic parts of the world (like Northern California), they can go together like diapers and wipes. An obstetrician from the Bay Area had this story about his oddest delivery.

I was born and raised in New Jersey. I got my first taste of medicine as a flight surgeon in the Pacific Theater. I thought I'd seen quite a bit by the time I finished my hitch in the service. But I'm living proof that you can still amaze the hell out of an old dog.

I guess it was two or three years before I retired. I'd helped deliver thousands of babies in my career. The guy I shared my practice with had a family emergency out of the country, so I had to fill his shoes and deal with a woman from the Bay Area. She was in her thirties, red-haired and seemed pretty average.

When they brought her in, she was just beginning labor. She had a guy with her, who may or may not have been the father—I learned early on never to ask or make any assumptions about the people who accompany pregnant women. Many a father has been mistaken for a grandfather, sisters for mothers and so on, so until I know the score, I keep the chatter light and minimal.

Well, this pudgy, white middle-aged guy was dressed in a grass skirt, with fringe on his wrists and ankles, what looked like tiger teeth on a string around his neck, wearing woven flip-flops and carrying a rattle capped by a shrunken skull. He looked like the Chief from King Kong's island. When I saw him, I could not contain myself and burst out laughing. And I just couldn't stop. I hadn't had a drink in two decades, but I felt like I'd been on a three-day bender and had just seen Queen Lizzie take a pie in the face. I laughed so long and so hard, the nurses became edgy. Of course, seeing their worried faces only made me laugh harder. I mean, there's this perfectly normal woman prepped for delivery, and standing by her side is this guy in an outfit unlike anything I'd ever seen. And then the woman says, "I don't see what's so funny. This is Allen, my shaman."

That doubled me over, and I was beginning to worry, because if I didn't stop laughing, I was certain to vomit. But every time I looked at Allen the Shaman, he blinked very slowly, kind of like a turtle trying to figure out a math problem, and that made me laugh more.

Now I was completely out of control. I was looking around the room, figuring Allen Funt must be mixed up in this somehow. Then Allen the Shaman makes a mean face and shakes the skull rattle at me. Well, that did it. I sprinted to the bathroom and threw up.

Maybe Allen really knew some witch doctoring, because the upchucking helped me put a lid on the yuks.

I cleaned myself up and got down to business. During her labor, the woman and Allen told me all about their pastiche of occult beliefs, which spanned the globe from Wicca to Feng Shui to Voodoo and everything in between.

At one point, Allen pulled out a fifth of Bacardi, a shot glass and a big green stogie from a gym bag. He poured a belt of rum and put it on the floor by the door with the cigar. "What's that for?" I asked him. "The Baron Samedi," he says. I've since learned that's some Voodoo demigod who looks like Charles Barkley in a top hat.

Allen didn't light the cigar or incense he brought, but at one point he sprinkled some protective dust around the bed. He had something he called an Apache healing drum. Looked to me like one of those noise-making trinkets with two little balls on strings they sell at Disneyland.

I don't know if Allen the Shaman's magic worked or not. I guess it didn't hurt, because the woman had a beautiful baby boy. And I got the laugh of my life, no question.

EXTRA! EXTRA! READ ALL ABOUT IT!

Maureen O'Boyle, who anchored EXTRA! through some of its biggest stories and highest ratings, opted to stay home and raise her daughter. A consummate pro, she gave birth and was still ready for her close-up.

$\mathcal{W}$e usually tape *EXTRA!* between noon and three, but if we have to re-tape something, we can go much later. On this day, everything was running late. I had a 3:00 doctor's appointment for a sonogram that I didn't want to miss. I'd canceled others before, but something told me it was really important to make this one.

It was close to 3:00 and I was sitting on the set getting ready to leave when we were told we needed to redo some takes. I started crying and everyone looked at me like I was a drama queen. "You don't understand, I *have* to make this appointment!"

Well, the doctor was able to juggle his schedule. As soon as we wrapped, I jumped in my car and zoomed through rush-hour traffic in the San Fernando Valley. I traveled from Burbank to Tarzana in record time.

As I weaved through the cars, I thought about the appointment. My doctor had been concerned that the baby hadn't gained enough weight. But I had followed his advice. During the last few weeks, I rested for four hours each day and five on the weekend. I put on extra weight. Everything has to be fine, I thought.

When the doctor put the sonogram wand on my stomach, it made this totally weird sound. I can't describe it, but it wasn't that *whoosh, whoosh, whoosh* noise I was used to. He looked up at me.

"I hope you don't have any dinner reservations tonight."

"What do you mean?"

"You're having a baby right now. We need to get this baby out right now." So I was out of his office, in my car and at the hospital, which was about a block away from the doctor, in minutes.

All of this was high drama for me, but it was very ordinary for the hospital. I couldn't get over how quiet it was. I walked down this long, soundless hall. A nurse calmly checked me in. I said, "Shouldn't people be rushing around, nervous and scared?"

The woman replied, "No. We do this every day. Many times a day."

I guess I've seen too many movies.

They put me in this little room and I started crying because my family's thousands of miles away and the baby's father was out of town. But I called everyone I knew in Los Angeles, and slowly but surely, my girlfriends started trickling in.

That's when I realized I was in full television makeup. And television makeup isn't something that just comes off with soap and water. Everyone who came in had a comment. "Wow, you look like you're going to your prom."

I said, "Hey, it's the first time my child's going to see me— I might as well look good."

Two of my friends were in the room as I had a C-section. The nurse told them to run their fingers through my hair to keep me calm. But their fingers kept getting caught in all the hair spray.

One of my friends said, "I don't know what I'm doing here. I faint at the sight of blood." Then, as the doctor opened me up, she said, "Cool. I can see all your insides!"

Even though I couldn't see anything, having my insides taken out was the most horrible sensation in my life. I kept saying, "Oh my God, it hurts!" My doctor would say, "It doesn't hurt, it's just really grossing you out. Don't think about it."

He was right—it didn't hurt. But just knowing what was going on seemed so scary and painful, I was having imaginary aches. But I forgot all about it when my 6-pound, 13-ounce daughter was placed on my chest. I couldn't believe it was a girl because I was convinced I was having a boy. Since I was on television, people would come up to me all the time and tell me I was having a boy. Total strangers would touch my stomach and say, "I've never been wrong about predicting the sex of a child, and you're definitely having a boy."

Keegan, the maiden name of my dad's mom, was so cute from the moment she was born. I loved her tremendously the first second I saw her. I loved her even more the next day and the next day. The whole thing is beyond words—she's a little miracle.

I still don't know why I needed an emergency C-section. Once the baby was born healthy and beautiful, I forgot to ask, "So what was the big problem?" I was too busy falling in love with her.

TAILGATE PARTY

Andrea, an executive from Winston-Salem, North Carolina, couldn't escape football, even when in labor.

*M*y husband, George, and I agree on most things, which is why our marriage has been pretty successful over the last fifteen years. The point where we diverge is sports, particularly football. I can't stand it! Everything about it bugs me—from the stupid rules to the fat-bellied referees in those too-tight shirts. What could be exciting about watching a bunch of supposedly grown men chase one another around a field—ugh!

But George loves it. Usually when there's a Sunday game that he has to see, I disappear with friends and get some shopping done. When we were first married, I actually tried to take an interest, but with eight or ten of his buddies on hand, I could tell I inhibited their fun. So I'd just get lost.

While I was pregnant with our first child, disappearing wasn't an option. I was huge and in no shape to go wander a mall for several hours while George and his apes swilled Heineken and threw Cheez Doodles at one another. So, I would just lock myself in a bedroom with a novel and my Walkman and try to tune out the game. One time, as I lay back, I was thinking, "Hey, this is pretty comfortable," when suddenly it felt like somebody whacked my back with a hammer. Not long after, a contraction ran through me. George had picked the wrong Sunday to host the game at our house.

I lay there and thought about it for a while. The birth class had said that you could delay for hours before heading to the hospital. Though I hate football, I love my husband. I figured, Let's just take it easy. Maybe he can finish the game. Besides, I really don't like hospitals.

I finished another chapter in my book, and then my water broke. I could not believe the volume of liquid that gushed out of me! I started getting contractions closer together. I waded to the bedroom door—the carpet was squishing between my toes.

"George!"

No answer, just the sounds of laughs and high fives. I was getting pissed. "GEOOOOOORGE!"

That time he heard me. When he came into the bedroom, he was cool. He grabbed my suitcase and I put on some dry clothes. As we walked out into the living room, he told the guys to enjoy the game and be sure to lock the door on the way out.

We got to the hospital and were checked right in. I was at three or four centimeters. The doctor showed up and said it would probably be a few hours. Then they gave me the epidural. I lay back and relaxed. Out of the corner of my eye, I thought I saw one of George's football buddies by the door to my room. I thought, I must be high.

George sat by my bed, talking. Then, from where I couldn't tell, I heard voices going, "Geoooorgie. Geoooorgie!" George's head snapped up. He looked out the window and started to laugh. I turned on my side and made him elevate the bed so I could see, too. Out in the parking lot, just below my window, his nutball pals had set up a tailgate party, and it was raging! And, as I looked, I realized that it was all stuff from my house. One of his pals had a mammoth pickup truck, and they had cold cuts and potato salad (in my bowls), a little charcoal barbecue with hot dogs and burgers, our portable television, my blender whirring away and, of course, a cooler full of beer. They were all laughing like hell and pointing and yelling, "Come on down here, boy!"

I could only shake my head. The nurse and the doctor laughed. George gave me his "please" look. He ran down there for a while—long enough to scarf down a dog and a beer, I guess, because when he returned, he smelled like both. After a while, somebody must have complained about the party, because they sicced security on them. Of course, somebody was pals with security, so they just had a hot dog and watched the game for a while, too.

I have to say, when the serious pushing started, George forgot all about his friends and was very attentive. When little Carol Ann came into the world (weighing 6 pounds, 14 ounces) he must have thrown a sign to his buddies, because we heard cheers and whoops from the parking lot.

Carol Ann is a wonderful little girl—she's very confident and always happy. I think it's because the first thing she ever heard was a cheer for her arrival.

CAN WE PUSH?

Melissa Rivers, who co-hosts the Oscar and Emmy fashion shows on E! Entertainment Television with her mother, Joan Rivers, held her mom's hand throughout her own labor.

*A*t thirty-seven weeks, the doctor discovered that I was running out of amniotic fluid. (I like to say that I was a quart low.) Anyway, he decided to induce me that week.

When I woke up on Thursday, November 30, I felt sick to my stomach. I assumed I was just really nervous since it was the morning of my inducement. I had about a million errands to run before I went to the hospital that night. I was all over town. Then that evening I met my mom, husband and in-laws for dinner. Afterward, I went to the hospital with my mom and John, my husband. That's when the doctor told me it hadn't been nerves at all. I'd been in labor all day. I was already a centimeter dilated!

At 10 P.M., they started inducing me. They estimated that the baby probably wouldn't be born for at least another twelve hours. We had plenty of time. My mom and my husband were both in the room and pretty soon they were out cold, snoozing on a pair of rocking-chair ottomans.

While they slept, I watched television. I'm a huge *Law & Order* fan, so I caught an episode. Then I clicked over to A&E for a while. We still didn't have a president, so I watched the news. At 2:30 A.M., I decided the pain was getting pretty strong and that an epidural was in order. I wanted John to hold my hand through the epidural, but he wouldn't wake up. I kept calling for him. "Honey. Honey. HONEY. WAKE UP!" I got the epidural and everything felt wonderful. I looked at John and said, "This is the best I've felt in months." I was in active labor, but it suddenly felt great.

A few seconds later, John fell back asleep. Then I dozed off.

But the nurses checked me every fifteen minutes because I wasn't progressing, and every half hour they rolled me over. I was in and out of sleep.

My mom had told me the story of my birth. She made it sound so easy that I felt I had a lot to live up to. She had been on stage performing when she felt her first stabs of labor pain. She even finished her act, went home, ate a sandwich and watched a movie. Then she fell asleep. The next morning she casually went to the doctor and had me a few hours later. No fuss, no muss. She said they gave her a little Demerol and she remembers nothing. When I ask her about it, she says it was very easy.

When I first started making plans for the birth, I knew my mom would want to stay in the room with us. She'd be too wound up and nervous to leave. But I told her, "I don't want you in there when I'm about to give birth. I don't need you to see me with my legs up in the air."

Mom and John were happily sleeping when I woke them up at 6:30 A.M. to tell them it was time. After remaining at just a few centimeters, I suddenly progressed to ten in what seemed like a matter of minutes. It was time to start pushing, but they took forever to wake up. "Get up. Get up," I kept yelling.

When they were finally semi-alert I ordered my mom and John to brush their teeth. John still makes fun of me for that, but I didn't want my mom and husband breathing on me with horrible morning breath. They were still half asleep, so they were like zombies just following my instructions. I brushed my teeth, too. I didn't want my child's first memory of Mommy to be bad breath.

I noticed Mom was still in the room. Instead of kicking her out, I turned to her and said, "Leave. Stay. Do what you want. I don't care. Just get out of the way." Then she was gone. A while later, I looked around and there she was, wedged behind the head of the bed. I have absolutely no idea how she did that. She was right over my face. I reached back and held her hand, which was really nice. She held my hand throughout the birth. We were both happy that she was standing where she was. "I had the perfect view," she tells people. She could only see what I could see—which was really nothing. Earlier, I had looked at the mirror near my legs and said, "Aaahhh! I can't watch this."

While I pushed, every now and then, I'd watch the *Today* show. We still didn't have a president.

At 7:30 A.M. on December 1, 2000, after an hour of pushing, little Edgar Cooper Endicott was born weighing 6 pounds, 15 ounces. I think the baby has my coloring and my big ol' lips. He's got a big round bowling ball of a head, just like my husband. John kept looking at the baby, saying, "Oh my God, this is a total miracle." My mother, of course, was crying.

I didn't cry then. But I practically did the first night in the hospital. They wheeled Coop into the room. His little hair was combed over to the side. He looked like an angel. But by four in the morning, he was a complete mess. John and I got up and pushed him back into the nursery. We had run out of bottles. He was crying and covered in formula. We were like, "Take him away!" Between the three of us, we had dismantled the bassinet. I was crying and John and my mom were about to cry. When we checked in on him at 6 A.M., though, he was back to being a little angel.

I know how to perform on cue. It's part of the job description, especially when you're working live. So I didn't scream or get hysterical during the birth. I just set my mind to the task at hand. But I'll tell you, I couldn't have done it without the epidural. It was also nice to have good old Mom in the room holding my hand. No matter how old you are, you always need your mommy. I hope Coop one day agrees.

HEY, HOT PANTS—WATCH THIS!

Anita from Hartford, Connecticut, decided to tame her
unruly daughter with a dose of delivery.

$\mathcal{B}$ob and I were shocked when we became pregnant
with our second child. We always wanted more kids, but had
thought it was impossible. After all, our only child was fifteen.

And what a handful! Jessica was out of control. She would go
to these crazy parties and come home while I'd be puking from
morning sickness. I know this is terrible to say about your kid, but
she was dressing like a little slut. She wore these tight, short skirts.
And the makeup! I swear she was beginning to look like a televangelist's wife. Of course, boys were showing up at our house like
horny dogs. They'd drive up, honk their horn and wait for Jessica
to run out in one of her hooker costumes.

One night I saw a pickup truck parked in front of the house
with the windows all steamed up. I spied from my bedroom as
Jessica finally stumbled out of the truck. Her blouse was untucked.
Her hair was a mess. She was so drunk she zigzagged up to our
front door.

I didn't say anything that night, but the next day I tried to talk
to her. I told her if she was having sex or planning to, she better
use birth control. One new baby in the family was enough. Jessica
said one new baby was too many. Then she stormed up to her
room and slammed the door.

My husband and I were pulling our hair out. Trying to battle
Jessica along with morning sickness and mood swings was too
much. I think I spent most of my pregnancy crying.

Then Bob had an idea.

"Why don't you invite Jessica into the delivery room?"

I was against it. I couldn't imagine my daughter seeing me naked
with my legs spread out in stirrups. Bob said something corny like

maybe we could all get closer through this birth. I knew what he was really thinking: Maybe if she saw how scary giving birth was, she'd think twice before letting some guy down her pants.

I went into labor at four in the morning. For the first time in months, Jessica was speaking to me. "What does it feel like?" Maybe Bob was right. Suddenly we felt like a family again.

The contractions were only a minute apart by the time I got to the hospital. They quickly wheeled me into the delivery room and examined me. This baby was coming fast. I was already completely dilated. I started pushing right away.

When I had Jessica I was nearly comatose from all the drugs they pumped into me. This time I decided to do it naturally.

"Oh my God, Mommy, are you okay?" Jessica looked scared. I guess she was so used to those cutesy births on television that she had no idea how much blood there really is.

Bob wiped my face with a compress. Then he whispered in my ear, "Don't be such a martyr. Why don't you scream a little? Let Jessie know how painful it is."

Another contraction hit me. I took a deep cleansing breath. Then I screamed as I pushed. I guess I yelled really loud because everyone in the room just stared at me with open mouths. Jessica looked horrified, so I screamed again—and again.

"Mom, stop it. Do you know how noisy you are?"

"Childbirth is fucking painful," I said. Jessica looked shocked. I'd never cursed in front of her before.

Another contraction hit me. "AHHH!!!!!!" Even though I was in pain, I was having some fun.

Bob whispered again, "Don't overdo it, honey."

I should have been an actress because I scared the crap out of Jessica. I knew she'd think about this moment the next time a boy honked his horn for her. Maybe I wouldn't be able to keep her a virgin, but she'd use about ten kinds of birth control. Believe me, this was better than any gourmet coffee moment with your daughter.

Our baby was a girl. We let Jessica cut the umbilical cord. I swear, the three of us just cried and cried as we stared at Anna. She was beautiful. She looked just like her sister did as a baby.

I was right. The childbirth experience worked magic. Jessica stays in many nights baby-sitting Anna. And when she does go out, she's home before midnight. She's even wearing longer skirts.

Who knows? Maybe I'll get a break for a while—or at least until my baby Anna becomes a teenager.

HOW MUCH WAS A MEZZANINE SEAT?

When *Melrose Place* vixen Josie Bissett and husband Rob Estes (*Melrose Place, Providence, Suddenly Susan*) decided to invite an audience into the delivery room, they never dreamed the drama would rival an episode of their TV show. Here's Josie's story:

I woke up at four in the morning with the feeling that something was about to happen. I reached over to feel for Rob, but he was gone. "Honey," I said. Rob answered from the floor. "I'm here."

Rob couldn't sleep and didn't want to wake me, so he moved to the floor. As we talked, I got the strangest sensation. "Honey, I think my water just broke." As I said this, water poured out of me. "My water did break."

We both started calling about a dozen friends and family members. We had decided early on that we wanted this birth to be shared with those closest to us. Our doctor knew and the hospital had accommodated us with extra chairs and a bigger room.

I'm also very into photo albums, so right away Rob started taking pictures. We wanted to document as many moments as possible. I figured one day I could present the album to my baby so he'd know what was going on before he was born. Even as we drove to the hospital, Rob snapped pictures of me. We were very calm.

When I got to the hospital, the labor pains became more and

more intense. I immediately asked for an epidural. I wanted to enjoy the birth as much as possible, and what's enjoyable when you're in pain?

Soon, friends and family started arriving, and I was feeling much better. My mother-in-law and sister-in-law got there first, followed by my sister and her kids. My parents arrived at around eight. It was a very festive atmosphere with people just filtering in like guests at a party. Besides me and the doctor and nurses, there were ten people in the room.

That's probably why the time went by so quickly. My family stayed with me the whole time. They only left when the doctors checked me. When I started pushing, Rob and I thought we'd ask everyone to leave except my mom and sister. But everything had been so easy. I dilated so quickly. We were shocked when it was time to push. Rob and I just sort of decided to let everyone stay in. Even my dad stayed in, but he was up by my head.

I'm really happy with that decision because it's such an amazing experience. I had seen my sister deliver her baby a few months earlier and there's nothing like watching someone give birth.

Rob was on one side, my sister-in-law on the other. Mom and Dad were up by my head. My sister videotaped while a friend took pictures. Everything seemed perfect.

Before I knew it, I was pushing in this room filled with all the people I love. Rob was an amazing coach. He counted to ten so loud and fast that the doctor had to keep telling him to slow down. I pushed for about an hour, but it went so fast. It seemed that it was only a few minutes later that 9-pound Mason Tru popped out. He was goopy and blue and beautiful. Everyone in the room was crying as the doctor lifted him up and put him on my chest.

My eight-year-old niece, Austin, stared in wonderment. I guess no one mentioned to her what the baby would look like when it came out. I think she sort of figured it would be all nice and clean, just like the movie babies.

I was in complete heaven. Then I turned toward Austin, who was up by my head, to show her the baby. As I smiled at her, her eyes rolled back and out she went. Next there was pandemonium. My sister screamed. My mom screamed at my dad to catch her. The doctor told them to lay her down. Someone else yelled that they should sit her up.

Then little Mason started choking from the fluid he swallowed. I was panicked. While chaos reigned, my child gasped for breath. I finally screamed, "Suction the baby! Suction the baby!"

All this hysteria probably lasted only a few seconds, but it seemed like a long time. My dad had caught Austin and she came to very quickly. Everyone laughed about it. Austin will always remember the day her cousin was born. And she has a great story for school.

3

Man, Thy Name Is Vanity...
and You, Too, Girls

Regardless of the situation, some people just have to look good.

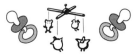

HEY, FRANK: JUST DO IT!

Jolene Ver Mulm, a mom from Prosser, Washington, had six children in six and a half years. No twins! While Frank, her husband, is a pretty normal guy, every time she heads into labor, he goes slightly nuts.

During the birth of Nick, my first son, I had to hold my arm straight up the entire time. I don't know why, but it seemed to help the pain. My husband stood next to the bed throughout the labor holding my left arm high in the air. At first he didn't complain, but after a few hours of this, his arm was really sore. I told him he couldn't let go—he thought his arm hurt, how did he think my whole body felt?

Anyway, everything worked out fine. Nick was healthy and beautiful. Only a little over a year later, I was in labor again. I was about four or five centimeters at my doctor's appointment, so they told me to check into the hospital around 1 P.M. We were biding our time, driving around. But as the time got closer and closer, I could tell Frank was getting a little nervous. Suddenly, he says, "Let's go to the furniture store."

We did need a couch and we still had some time before the appointment. Besides, there were plenty of chairs and sofas I could sit on and, most important, there was a bathroom. So we just wandered around, looking at sofas. We didn't find anything we liked. My contractions were not that serious, but every now and then, I'd have to bend over against a sofa for the pain.

Finally we head for the car. Frank starts driving. After a few minutes I realize we're not anywhere near the hospital. It's closer to our appointment and my contractions are getting stronger. As calmly as possible, I ask Frank, "Where are we going?"

Well, he turns into the Big 5, which is a sporting goods chain. He sort of looks at me sheepishly. "I just need to make a quick stop."

"What for?"

"If I have to stand for hours holding up your arm again, I need some new shoes. These are killing my feet!"

As you can imagine, I was shocked. I was worried about more than sore feet at the moment. But I did know my body. It kind of fiddled around for a while during labor, so I thought we had a little time. Frank and I went into the store.

Soon I was breathing through pretty serious contractions. Frank was trying on one pair of sneakers after another. The contractions are stabbing at me so I'm leaning over benches trying to deal with the pain. My eyes are squeezed shut. I may have been moaning a bit. When the contraction passes, I look around. People are staring at me. Everyone looked pretty nervous. I think they thought I was going to give birth to the baby right in the store.

Frank, of course, is oblivious. He's still trying on sneakers. There was a waist-high drift of rejected footgear piled up next to him. They make running shoes, walking shoes, sneakers for aerobics, basketball, baseball and tennis. Nothing seemed to fit right. Too bad Nike doesn't have a line of labor-room sneaks. I told

Frank we had to get moving. He settled on a pair and headed for the checkout line. By then, I was nearly doubled over in pain.

As we wait, I can tell something else is on Frank's mind. I know he wants to ask me something. He turns to me and says quickly, "I need a new shirt."

I am beside myself. We'd already been in the store for forty-five minutes. "What for? That shirt is fine, but I'm not!"

"Yeah, but I wore the same shirt when Nick was born."

"SO WHAT'S THE BIG DEAL?"

"Well, I'll have the same shirt on in the pictures."

"Who cares? We're going!"

Frank didn't argue. We headed to the hospital and Elle, our daughter, was born in two hours, weighing 8 pounds, ½ ounce. Now that I've had a few more, I know that walking around was probably the best thing for me: If I'd gone to the hospital they would have put me in bed. It was better for me to be distracted by my husband's craziness. Maybe he knew something I didn't.

Nah.

After three births in the hospital, we decided to try home birthing. For the day of the delivery, the doctor instructed Frank to put a plastic sheet on the bed. Instead, Frank put plastic on the bed, halfway up the walls, into the halls and through the bathroom. The doctor came in, took one look around and said, "Frank, this is insane! We gonna have a baby or mud wrestle?"

Frank goes, "Well, you've never seen my wife have babies. It can be kind of scary. Things just fly out everywhere." Our daughter, Elle, shot out like a cannonball. The doctor had to catch her by the foot. I think that's the picture Frank still had in his mind and it terrified him.

This was all a coping technique for Frank. But by now he's an old pro. For baby number five, Frank didn't have to hold my arm up—our four-year-old did!

I was thankful to be at home for this birth. The whole family was watching a movie while I was breathing through contractions. My two-year-old looked at my face and announced, "Everyone be quiet, Mommy is having tractors."

A few days after the birth, our five-year-old ran to Daddy and squealed, "The most exciting thing happened today—the baby's extension cord fell off."

By the time number six arrived, there wasn't any plastic or new shoes or trips to the furniture store. Nick even helped his daddy cut the umbilical cord. I think Frank might have had the same shirt on, but with so many kids he didn't notice.

Now it's a house filled with children and love and a touch of craziness. We gave each child a four-letter name—Nick, Elle, Hidi, Hani, Hali and Levi. I had no idea we'd have so many children, but all their names fit on our Christmas card. The children look so much alike. Friends of ours have commented, "Another batch, but the same recipe."

It's a pretty great recipe.

THE QUICK-CHANGE ARTIST

Abby, a labor nurse from Los Angeles, California, told this tale of ego, pomposity and just plain weirdness.

This couple was very nice, but the guy seemed really nervous. They came into the hospital at about 3 P.M. on a Saturday. They were a typical yuppie couple, casually dressed for a backyard barbecue or something.

She was already at about five or six centimeters, so we got her right into the delivery room. Matt, the husband, paced around and checked his watch. I wanted to ask him if he had an appointment somewhere.

After about forty-five minutes, the mother was at eight centimeters—only two more and she'd be completely dilated. At that point, I explained, it would be time to start pushing.

"When will that be?" asked Matt.

I told him it could be pretty soon.

"I have to run out for a few minutes," he told me.

I said that if he needed a camera, the gift shop sold disposables that were pretty good. He really didn't answer me one way or another. Between breaths, his wife asked him what was wrong.

"Nothing . . . I just need to go home for a few minutes," he told her.

She wailed, "If you leave you might miss everything!" Then she sort of nodded to me like, Will you confirm that arrival is imminent?

"What time will it be born?" asked Matt.

The doctor said, "I can't say exactly. Might be fifteen minutes, might be two hours or more."

With that, Mr. Nervous is out the door like a shot. Twenty minutes later, his baby daughter is born. A half hour later, the baby's all cleaned up and cuddling with Momma. In walked Matt, in a three-piece suit.

"Where the hell were you? And what are you wearing?"

"I had to go home and change. I didn't want my child's first impression of me to be a guy in a polo shirt and khakis."

He was serious! What a nut!

HIS COLORS WERE COORDINATED, RIGHT?

As a labor nurse for nearly two years, Melanie Lemen of Cleves, Ohio, thought she knew all there was about birthing babies. That is, until she had her own.

It's all about feet. When you work in labor and delivery, you really notice every foot up there in the stirrups. And so many women have horrible feet. Smelly. Scaly. Feet with twisted nails. Feet with warts. Feet with fungus. Most of these women haven't been able to see their feet in months, so they have no idea how disgusting they have become.

Then there are the women who have to wear their lucky socks. They'll be smelly and filthy with black bottoms, but somehow they're lucky. Maybe because they keep everyone away! As a labor nurse, I wound up spending a lot of time with my nose next to women's feet. I was really sensitive about it when I was getting close to delivering.

I had told my doctor about this foot fetish. When I had my weekly appointment, he said, "You're starting to dilate. You better get your pedicure before this baby comes." So I went right in for a pedicure. This was October so I had my toenails painted in a warm tone–burgundy. I have to say, my feet looked great and they felt so soft. I was ready to go.

On Saturday, a few days later, I started getting contractions. They were pretty strong and close together. It was the football season, so Brad, my husband, with his face glued to the television, said, "If you're in labor by the end of the third quarter, we'll go." We waited and then called my doctor, who said, "Come in right away."

I had started bleeding, too, so I was a little frantic. I had packed my bag days before. I just wanted to get to the hospital as fast as possible to see the baby on the monitor, to be reassured that everything was fine.

I thought Brad had gone outside to bring the car around. While I waited, I called my mom. I was so excited. Then I headed for the door.

But the car wasn't there. I waited and waited. Minutes went by–still no Brad. On a hunch, I walked into the bedroom, and there he was, standing in the closet looking at his clothes. He looked completely panicked.

"I don't know what to wear."

I couldn't believe it! Brad is never fussy about clothes. His uniform usually consists of jeans and any old T-shirt.

"Let's go," I said.

"I just want to look nice," he said. "I can't be all rough and rugged when I'm meeting the baby for the first time."

He's putting shirts on and pulling them off. He's holding up different shirts against his chest.

I couldn't believe it! He wanted to make a good first impression. What was he thinking? Was the baby going to look at him and say, "Gee, Daddy, you really know how to put yourself together! Now change my diaper, you handsome devil."

Brad was still holding shirts up against himself when I grabbed some clothes, shoved them in his face and said, "You're wearing this!" It was a sweater vest and a pair of jeans. I was ready to kill him.

We got to the hospital at 9:30 that evening. The nurse said, "She's five to six centimeters dilated," and I was like, "Woo-hoo, I'm in labor!" I got an epidural around midnight and rested through the night. Brad and I even fell asleep for a while. At about 7 A.M., I started pushing.

My doctor looked at me and said, "Oh, Melanie, you're going to be disappointed, but I have to put a drape over your feet. Your nice pedicure isn't going to show up in the pictures." At one point, he was going to cut holes in the sheet but decided it wouldn't be very sterile. So my burgundy toes didn't make it into any pictures, although I knew my feet sure looked great in the stirrups.

Brad and I called tons of people. We phoned Brad's family and my family. The nurses and doctors really laughed because in the middle of a push, I'd command Brad to call my mom, who was in St. Louis and couldn't get there in time. I'd get on the phone with my mom and say, "Mom, I can see some hair now." Then I'd hear her pass the news on to the rest of the family who had gathered there. "She can see the hair." I'd push again and give another update.

At 9:47 A.M. on October 17, Caroline was born weighing 7 pounds, 15 ounces. Everything about her was perfect. The entire birthing experience was wonderful.

Whenever a friend is pregnant, I offer only two pieces of advice. I say, "Make sure you get your toenails done. It feels really good and the doctor will really appreciate it." Then I tell them to make sure their husbands know what they're going to wear to the hospital. I guarantee it will be their fault if you're late for your child's birth.

WOW! LOOK AT THAT REAR END!

Theresa, a travel writer from New York, and her husband, Joe, a television executive, gave birth to a surprisingly massive (11-pound) baby boy. As Mom tells it . . .

*W*hen we got to the hospital, I wanted Joe to sneak me in through a service entrance because my weight had zoomed by nearly fifty percent. "Good idea," he said. "The doors are probably wider, too." I wanted to split his head with a pipe wrench.

First they put me in a triage unit. Then, when I reached five centimeters, they took us up to a delivery room. The place surprised me—it had soft lights, a normal-looking bed and a big reclining chair. Joe flopped in the chair as if it were in our living room.

After a while, things started heating up, the contractions got closer and stronger and the pain got worse. The anesthesiologist was summoned and gave me an epidural. In a few minutes I felt like I was at a cocktail party. La la la!

Twelve hours later, it just wasn't happening. They decided a cesarean was in order. Suddenly, Joe's in full scrubs looking like an extra from *Chicago Hope* and there's hospital personnel swarming around me like I'm writing free malpractice policies.

Joe, clown that he is, started laughing and barking orders at no one in particular. "Suction!" "Forceps!" "Ten cc's of Framazine!" I always knew he was insane, but what a time to clown it up! The surgical team was looking at him like he was out of his skull, and I was getting plenty of pity stares.

I was *so* embarrassed about my weight, especially my rear end. I figured about sixty pounds had settled in my caboose. As the doctor cut me, a tubby nurse shouted, "Wow, look at that rear end!" Joe laughed hysterically.

"You're not exactly Kate Moss yourself, honey," I answered.

"I'm referring to your baby, ma'am," she replied curtly.

"Ma'am." I hate "ma'am." In bitch-ese, "ma'am" means "fuck you."

When they cut me, the baby was rump-side up, so he came out mooning everyone. When they put him on my chest, I couldn't believe how massive he was.

When they brought me down to a regular room, Joe was still in his scrubs. He kept darting in and out of my room, wandering around the hospital, digging it every time someone mistook him for a doctor. He claimed he even walked into some woman's room, read her chart and asked her how she was feeling today. He signed her chart "Marcus Welby."

My freak of a husband. My fat-bottomed baby. What a day!

SO, DID YOU SLIP HIM YOUR NUMBER LATER?

Cara, a mom from Denver, Colorado, always hoped she'd run into her first love. Just not on a bad butt day. The doctor's name has been changed to protect the innocent.

I'm in the delivery room a few centimeters dilated when one of the nurses asks me if I want an epidural. I'm no martyr. I don't believe in pain, so I say yes. The nurse smiles and tells me she's going to page Dr. Scott Ainsley, the anesthesiologist. "Don't worry, he'll be here in a few moments," she says.

Dr. Scott Ainsley! I couldn't believe it. He was my high school sweetheart! My first boyfriend. And here I am. My fat ass hanging in the air. Fifty pounds overweight. My face covered with some weird pregnancy acne. "Is he the only anesthesiologist available?" I ask. Yes, they tell me.

I'm in searing pain. My insides are on fire. I can't stand it. But I also can't imagine the thought of Scott in here. It's too much. Sure, I know, he's seen hundreds of women just like me. But he broke my heart. If he's gonna see me, it's gonna be when I look hot. Just like I'd imagined in all my revenge fantasies.

"You know what? I'm going to try to do this naturally," I blurt. I grit my teeth and stifle a scream as a contraction plows through me. My husband's mouth hangs open for about five minutes.

The pain was beyond horrible. But I got through it knowing the alternative was much, much worse.

4

Florence Nightingale . . . Not!

Here're some people whose bedside manner leaves much to be desired.

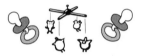

NEXT TIME, SPRITZ HIM WITH BIMBO REPELLENT

Linda, an insurance executive from Los Angeles, California, learned that even her baby's birth wasn't going to keep the women away from her trophy husband.

$\mathcal{M}$y husband is an actor. A very, very good-looking actor. I love him like crazy, but sometimes I wish he weren't always so incredibly hot. And what makes him extra, extra sexy and attractive is he has no idea just how good-looking he is. So women swarm him like flies. And his wedding ring means nothing to them. If anything, I think it just heightens the challenge factor.

He can be anywhere—waiting for an elevator, in line for a taco, putting gas in the car—and women will come up to him and hit on him. Many offer their phone numbers. One time at a gas station, some pushy bitch was really hitting on him hard. When he went inside to pay, she left her phone number under his windshield wiper—wrapped in a condom! He thought this was pretty funny.

Just to get back at her, I made sure we used the condom right away. And then *I* used her phone number—dialing her and hanging up in the middle of the night, several times. I figured a couple of fat bags under her eyes might give her something to think about besides other women's husbands.

When my water broke, at about 3 A.M., we drove to the hospital without incident and were checked in immediately. It must have been a slow night, because everything seemed calm and quiet. We sat around watching the junky television you get at that hour. Mike kept channel-surfing, hoping to catch himself in a commercial he was appearing in.

Around 7 A.M., the nurses' shift changed. The nice, plump, middle-aged woman who had been checking on me wished me luck, and a few minutes later, in swung this Hollywood blonde who's all teeth and boobs. She must have had her little white uniform specially made of spandex—it fit that tight. She eyeballed my husband, and her face looked like a cat spotting a crippled robin. I'm thinking, Great—here we go!

Now, I'm not unattractive myself. But I put on forty pounds for the baby, haven't so much as walked around the block in nine months and I'm pretty certain I won't be approached by *Victoria's Secret* anytime soon.

When Miss TNT checked me, I wanted to slap her hand. Then she didn't even tell me how many centimeters I am or anything. She just swung her ass in my face and said to Mike, "Are you an actor?"

Well, Miss TNT kept up the pickup chatter. "I know I've seen you in movies. What have you done? You have that total Brad Pitt thing going." I figured any minute she's going to measure his inseam. I started looking around my bed, hoping to find a nice, heavy machine I could "accidentally" tip over onto her peroxide-soaked skull.

After a while, she was called to another room. Mike could see I was getting pissed. Of course, he always thinks these bimbos are just "being friendly" or polite. I yelled, "If she's so friendly and polite, why is she ignoring me—I'm having a baby here!"

She came back in, peeked under my sheet and squealed, "Ooh!

I better get a doctor!" My contractions were hurting a lot more, so they gave me something—I think it was called Stadol, or something like that. Even though I was in severe pain, I was thinking, "If I let them zonk me, this bitch will close in for the kill!" Then a searing pain hit, and I thought, To hell with it. She can have him. I want some relief.

Since I was slightly high from the drugs, I'll never be absolutely sure, but it seemed like Miss TNT kept brushing her Wonderbra'd boobs against Mike's arm, or bumping him with her ass as she worked around me. Of course, she was sneaky enough to do it very subtly, but I'm certain those body-part collisions were not in error.

When it came time for the heavy pushing, I was pretty distracted, but I did notice she kept staring at him. The next thing I knew, my baby was born and the pain ended. Mike was kissing my face and telling me how proud of me he was. Miss TNT put my squirming baby on my chest and said, "Here's your baby . . . he's beautiful—just like his daddy." And she winked at me!

I didn't care. I had my baby. And my husband. They're both beautiful. And *mine*. And if Miss TNT ever has a baby and decides to nurse it, I hope it likes the feel and taste of silicone!

YOU SEE, NURSES DON'T HAVE TO TAKE THE HIPPOCRATIC OATH

Durenda Wilson is a mother of six from Burlington, Washington. She had this story filled with action, adventure and a surprising twist.

I had a scheduled C-section for my second baby on New Year's Eve. At this time of year out here in Burlington, it's usually fifty-five and rainy. But that year we were caught by surprise with a cold snap and snow. Our Isuzu Trooper had four-wheel drive, so we thought we were fine. What could go wrong?

We're up really early for our 5:30 A.M. hospital check-in. Actually, I had tossed and turned the entire night, but I am running on adrenaline. Soon, though, we're in the car and heading the one and a half miles to the hospital.

We're cruising along trying to make it up a steep hill when one of our wheels freezes up. Before we realized that we're operating on three-wheel drive, our car spins out of control. On one side of us there's a cliff with a fifty-foot drop—on the other side is a ditch. It happened so fast, but we started praying. Our prayers worked because instead of plunging down the cliff, the tail end of the car skids right into the ditch. Darryl, my husband, guns the engine, but there's no way this car is going anywhere. We're stuck.

Next, I'm behind the wheel and Darryl's outside trying to push the car. He's yelling, "Okay, honey, gun it! Gun it!" I do, but I know we're not going anywhere. I turn around and see that he's completely covered in the mud spitting off the tires. "Gun it," he says again and again.

"Honey, you're covered in mud."

"It doesn't matter! Gun it again!"

After a few more all-out shoves, he accepts that we're not driving anywhere and decides to walk the half mile back to the house to get a neighbor. I'm sitting in the car with the engine running and the heat on. The road is deserted, but a few minutes after Darryl leaves, a car drives by. I'm thinking, This car will stop and help us. I mean, how could somebody see an occupied car stuck in a ditch and not stop to offer some assistance?

They drive right by. Where could they be going that is so important? After what seems like an eternity, Darryl and my neighbor return. Our neighbor couldn't stop laughing. He thought our whole predicament was hilarious. My husband had changed his clothes. And he wasn't laughing.

We're an hour late for the C-section. These two surgical nurses greeted me by saying, "You're late." A C-section is planned right down to the minute, so being late throws off a lot of people's schedules. They don't like tardiness when they have all the post-op people waiting for you.

I start to explain what happened. "Sorry, but we got stuck in a ditch."

As soon as the words leave my mouth the nurses simultaneously say, "What? That was you?"

My mouth hangs open. They had driven right by me!

I'm incredulous. "Why didn't you stop?"

They say in unison, "We were late for work."

"Ha! I was your work!"

I couldn't believe these two women were the surgical nurses. Now I'm thinking, Gee, if something goes wrong, I hope it doesn't happen during their coffee break. But little Jenna came out fine, weighing exactly 6 pounds.

I've been to the hospital for four more babies since then, and every time someone says, "Weren't you the woman who drove into a ditch?"

THE MONSTER-IN-LAW

Jenny from St. Louis, Missouri, wins the award for having the mother-in-law from hell.

I had been in labor for eighteen hours. The pain was intense. I didn't think things could get worse. And then my mother-in-law barged into the room.

She took one look at me—splayed out on the table, covered in sweat, gasping for relief—and Marge did what she does best: criticize.

"Oh my God, she's so swollen. Is that normal? When I had my Billy here, I never ballooned like that. Could this be serious? I saw an episode of *ER* just like this and the patient died in childbirth. Could that be what Jenny has? It's just not natural."

Marge was one of those annoying creatures who thought she knew absolutely everything there was to know. She'd done some volunteering as a candy striper, which meant she handed forms to patients at the check-in desk and rang up purchases in the gift shop. But in her mind, she was head of surgery.

"There's no difference between what I do and what they do. I even assisted in an appendectomy," Marge liked to say. Yeah, she held a door open for the doctor.

Marge was also an *ER* freak. I'd seen her shout at the television like a guy watching a football game. "Clamp it! Come on, scalpel! Code blue! Code blue! You're losing him!"

So while I was in labor, Marge played doctor. She put her hands on her hips, surveyed the delivery room and announced, "We'll have this baby out of you soon, but you need to really push. Bear down like you mean it. You don't know how to push. Let's exert a little energy, honey. Watch me."

She swallowed a ton of air. Then she tucked her chin into her neck and held her breath. Her face turned purple. She let out this long exhale.

"That's how you do it, honey. Billy, here, just slid out of me. But things were different then. When I was your age, I'd already had all six of my children. You wait so long these days. I told Billy you should have had kids years ago. But you all want careers. In my day, children were a career."

I couldn't take it anymore. I asked for more painkillers. As the doctor instructed the nurse to summon the anesthesiologist, Marge whispered to him, "She doesn't mean what she says. Jenny doesn't really want drugs."

"YES I DO!" I screamed.

"I won't have my grandchild born on drugs!"

"SHUT UP!"

Marge gasped. "I know that's the pain talking, Jenny dear. But you don't need drugs. I did it naturally, and look at my kids. There's not a druggie in the lot of them. You can do it, Jenny."

I felt the strongest urge to push. And kill.

"That's it, Jenny. You're almost there," the labor nurse said.

The doctor put on his gloves and moved in between the stirrups. I squeezed my eyes shut and pushed as hard as I could.

When I opened them, I saw Marge standing between the stirrups with forceps in hand.

"Here, take these before you let the head slip back again," she told the doctor.

"Get her out of my delivery room!" the doctor bellowed.

I don't think she was in the room when the baby was born, but she must have sneaked back in shortly after. Over my newborn's cries, I heard Marge say, "She's beautiful. I don't see any of Jenny in her."

THE SHIRTS ARE TERRIBLE, BUT THE BIRTHING PANTS WORK!

Casey Williams-Krubiner is a stand-up comedian and a mom from Toluca Lake, California, who offers her take on snoring husbands and nursing shirts.

*N*o one believed me when my water broke. I was at the hospital to be induced and they inserted this gel up me. Well, a few minutes later I feel this gush. I tell a nurse, "I think my water just broke." She gives me a know-it-all look and informs me that it's just the gel melting. They tell me to go home and come back later, but I'm feeling kinda weird. There's so much water and I'm in some pain. My husband's freaking out a bit. Finally, I convince a nurse to check me. She's like, "Oh yeah. Your water broke." They admit me.

By now it's 4:30 P.M. and I'm absolutely starving. I hadn't eaten since ten in the morning and none of the nurses would give me food. They say it's absolutely not allowed. I complain to a doctor who says of course I can eat something. Well, they bring me this turkey sandwich and to this day I consider it the best sandwich I've ever eaten. I was so hungry and this hospital meal suddenly tasted like gourmet food. Life is good. I'm so happy. A nurse comes in and asks me if I want an epidural.

"Nah. I'm not so bad," I say.

"You will be and you don't want to miss out," she tells me.

The doctor was passing through and he pokes his head in and goes, "Oh yeah, why don't you have it now?"

It's December 1, and as I wait for the epidural, I watch *Rudolph the Red-Nosed Reindeer*. Knowing I'm about to get pain relief triggers intense pain. Suddenly, I can't wait for the epidural, even though a few minutes ago I didn't want it. I'm staring at poor Rudolph as he's being teased for his red nose. He can't join in any reindeer games. Boo hoo! He thinks he has problems! What a wimp.

The epidural was the most horrible part of the whole delivery. I had no idea that it would take fifteen minutes for them to put that mile-long needle in your back. Then they demand you stay still. But you're having contractions, so it's nearly impossible not to move. When it's over I feel a lot better. The doctor tells me to try to sleep because this baby won't arrive until the morning.

I'm feeling tired and numb. Just as I start nodding off, my husband begins snoring.

Let me explain: My husband doesn't just snore, he conjures thunderstorms through his nasal passages. At home, I have a routine. If I go to sleep before him, his snoring won't wake me up. Once I'm asleep, nothing gets me. But now . . .

He's out cold on the reclining chair next to me. I'm going, "Honey. HONEY. HONEY!!" I try to punch him, but I can't move. I'm immobile from the waist down due to the epidural. I've got nothing to throw at him, either. He's just blissfully sawing away.

At 5 A.M., he wakes up and the nurses check me. I feel the baby pushing. I'm saying, "I think it's time." And the nurses smile and then nervously check their watches. I think they were under strict orders not to wake the doctor until 7 A.M. By 6, my husband's freaking out. The nurse tells me I can start pushing if I want to, but she's doing paperwork in another section of the room. I'm pushing and my husband is helping me. We didn't know what we were doing. At 7:05 the doctor breezes in.

My baby was born at 7:13 A.M. on December 2, 1999. I'm convinced that if the doctor had come earlier, she would have been born at about 5 A.M. But hey, you wouldn't want to deprive a doctor of a good eight hours.

We named her Lucy. I'm a comedian, so everyone assumes it's after Lucille Ball. But my real idol is Lucy Van Pelt, from *Peanuts*. Ever since I can remember, I always said I'd have a daughter named Lucy. I think Michael wanted me to consider other names. I kinda did, but there was never much chance I'd waver. I knew he'd eventually come around. It doesn't matter though. For some reason everyone calls her Smoopy. Don't ask.

Breast-feeding was a huge challenge for me, but it finally worked out. I had enough material to perform a whole comedy routine on nursing because so much of it is absurd. For instance, before I had Lucy, I bought a whole bunch of nursing tops because everyone says they're an absolute necessity. You just don't question the authorities. But you know what? You're more exposed than if you're wearing a regular shirt. Instead of just lifting your shirt up, you stick your boob through a huge hole in the middle of a shirt. Yeah, that's real subtle. But those "baby experts" get us naïve mothers with the nursing-shirt scam. Now that I know better, that's my advice to expectant moms: Don't fall for the nursing shirts!

THE PARKING SPOT

Nora, a mom from the San Fernando Valley, thought labor pains would be the scariest part of childbirth. Was she in for a surprise!

"Hello, I'm Marlys, and I'll be taking over for the night nurse. We'll be together for the duration of your labor and delivery."

A chill tore through me as my heart pounded. My husband shook her hand, introduced us and blabbered on about how happy he was to meet her.

As he gabbed, Marlys studied me.

"Did you have another child with me? You look sort of familiar."

I was about to say, "Yes, Marlys, that's it." Instead, my big-mouthed *in*significant other chimed in.

"No, this is our first child. And any advice you can give us would be great. We missed the last Lamaze session."

Marlys was relentless. "You do look familiar."

"Maybe you live near us," my idiot life partner offered.

Of course she lives near us, I wanted to scream at him. As a matter of fact, just a few months ago, Marlys and I nearly killed each other over a parking space.

It was a simmering August day. I was five months and change pregnant. I'd already gained twenty-five pounds. My back hurt. My hemorrhoids burned. I had indigestion. And there it was— a spot right in front of the supermarket. I was at the other end of the lane and I put my blinker on to claim it. That's the way it works in a civilized society. But Marlys turned into the lane from the other side and careened into the spot, like a vulture. My blinker clicked impotently.

I honked. Marlys ignored me. I honked again. Marlys exited the car and hit the door-lock button on her key chain. The car *beep-beeped,* mocking me. And Marlys headed toward the super-market as if she were oblivious to the entire event.

I rolled down my window. "Excuse me, that was *my* parking spot. I was waiting for it."

Marlys stiffened. She sneered as she turned toward me as if I were some drunken bum begging bus fare. She growled: "But I got there first."

I was furious. This witch practically admitted she had stolen the spot. Maybe she felt okay about it, but I needed her to be aware of certain things.

"Maybe you think it's all right to steal spots, but I just thought

I'd mention that I'm very pregnant and maybe next time you'll . . ."

Marlys marched over to my car and nearly stuck her face into the driver's window. Her narrow eyes blazed.

"I am so sick of pregnant women thinking the world owes them something. I've been pregnant, too, sweetheart, and I didn't expect the world to bow before me. All you pregnant women do is whine and complain. I can't stand any of you." Then she smiled a psycho smile.

"Besides, walking's good exercise."

I wanted to punch her face.

"You look like the one who could use some exercise."

Marlys, who was about forty pounds overweight, hissed through her teeth. "It's a thyroid problem, you bitch."

Bitch! How dare she call a woman carrying life a bitch!

"Thyroid problem? Is that what causes a fat ass?"

Then I sped home. I sent my husband to the supermarket later that evening.

That was nearly four months ago. I tried to remember what I was wearing. Maybe I had on my baseball cap and sunglasses. Maybe she won't recognize me now.

While Marlys checked the monitors hooked up to me, I whispered to my husband, "That nurse hates pregnant women."

He laughed and said, "I think the drugs are making my wife paranoid. Is that normal?"

I couldn't believe the idiot I married.

"Shut up," I said.

Marlys laughed and said, "You'll be hearing a lot worse before this is over. You wouldn't believe the things women tell their husbands when they're in this state."

Marlys inserted an intravenous needle in my arm. I was convinced it was dripping arsenic into my veins. The world around me spun.

"I want another nurse," I screamed.

My husband was mortified. He hates conflict and wants everyone to be friends. "Honey, Marlys is great," he told me. He turned to Marlys. "She's not usually like this. It must be the drugs and pain. Please forgive her."

Marlys winked at my husband. "Don't worry about it, honey. Pregnant women say the darnedest things. I could write a book."

The last needle kicked in, and Marlys was becoming a blur. Since no one would listen to me, I inhaled and exhaled and pushed. I prayed that Marlys wouldn't murder me. And if she had to kill me, I prayed that she would spare my child. Two hours later, baby Christopher was pulled out of me. The minute he emerged, all my paranoia disappeared. I realized Marlys had no idea who I was. I almost wanted to hug her for helping deliver this beautiful, wailing baby boy.

When Marlys placed my baby on my chest, she smiled wryly. "Mind if he parks in this space?"

THE PITCH

Margaret McCabe was delivering her firstborn in a hospital in Los Angeles, when her labor nurse decided to go Hollywood.

I told the labor nurse my husband was overseas directing a feature film. Her eyes lit up like halogens and she began to chatter like a magpie. I figured I knew what was coming—she had a screenplay.

"Hey, I'm just a housewife. I wouldn't know a good screenplay from a good football play," I offered. But she wasn't buying it; she was selling—hard. The next thing from her mouth was "Fade In." It really wouldn't have bugged me that much, but her nutty story was one of those teenage ax-in-the-face movies.

Originally from Lubbock, Jan had a Texas twang that made everything sound twice as gory—and annoying.

"So theyn, this little bitch in a belly shirt comes burstin' outta the closet swingin a bootcher knaahfe, an chaysuz Cindy 'roun 'n'

roun the beyd screamin' 'I'm gonna cut yew in a millyun pieces!'–
lessee, yore at about tayun cennameters–yore gonna hafta start
pushin' soon, honey . . ."

At the Harris Method birthing class, I'd been taught to think
calm, lovely thoughts to keep the pain at bay. My mental movie
was of me sitting in a little red wagon, being pulled through a field
of daisies and butterflies on a perfect summer day. Instead, I'm
getting "bootcher knahves and belly shirts."

"Okeye, now I need a real biyug push as Ahm countin' t'
tayun," directed Jan. I took a manatee-sized breath and pushed . . .

"Wuhn, two, thuh-ree, fower, faahve . . . now out in the parkin'
lot, Tiffany–that's the little bitch in the belly shirt–catches up to
Cindy and jes hacks a big ol' chunk a' flesh raaaht outa the side a'
her neck . . . heyull, did Ah lose count?"

I started praying for deliverance. Actually, Jan could have
been an extra in the film *Deliverance*. I had known birthing
wouldn't be easy, but this woman made it unbearable. Just at the
moment where I was about to grab the phone and call . . . who?
The cops? Mom? To say what? This labor nurse is a friggin'
nitwit and her gory screenplay is making me sicker . . . in walked
my OB/GYN.

"So, zero hour is nigh," he said.

"Can I have a word with you . . . in private?" I asked.

Jan knew what was coming and looked at me like she was audi-
tioning for the role of Tiffany–her eyes drilled me with 10,000-
watt hate beams. I wondered what was under her scrubs–a belly
shirt an' a bootcher knaahfe? The doctor nodded at her and she
left the room.

"What's wrong?" he asked with all the sincerity he could
muster.

"That labor nurse . . . I'm sure she's very competent, but she
insists on pitching me . . ."

"*Blood on the Lawn*? The screenplay?" He looked furious.

"Is that the title?"

Shaking his head, he picked up the phone and ordered another nurse to the room. My little baby boy, Alex, was born a few minutes later.

They put me in a private room overnight. I never slept a wink, worrying about a visit from Jan. And I insisted on nursing Alex every hour on the hour, for fear Jan might pay him a call.

5

Eeeeeewwwwww!

Do not, repeat, DO NOT attempt to read this chapter while eating.

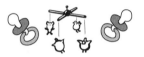

WARNING: UNIDENTIFIED FLYING PLACENTA

Carol Lynch from Metairie, Louisiana, was just following doctor's orders when . . .

I was on the phone with a friend when I started leaking. I said to her, "Gee, I can't even hold my pee anymore. I'm completely incontinent." This continued for a few hours before it dawned on me that perhaps my bag of waters had broken. I called the hospital and they said, "Get in here now."

David, my husband, and I got to the hospital at about 1 P.M. The doctor checked me and said, "Not much is going on." Not much went on for an entire day. While I waited and waited, all I wanted was back rubs. But I kept telling David he wasn't rubbing my back low enough. He said, "You don't want me to rub your back, you want me to rub your butt. Just say it." I said, "That's right. I want a butt massage, okay?"

After nearly a day of labor pains and butt massages, the contractions went from tolerable to excruciating. I started pacing the floor and contracting every seven steps. I'd stop and go,

"ARRRRRRRRRGGGGGGGGGGGGGH!" The nurse came in and asked, "What are you doing?" I said, "I don't know what the hell I'm doing. I'm in pain! I'm in a lot of pain."

"Maybe she's nearly dilated," David suggested.

The nurse checked me and then looked at us strangely. "Oh honey, you are not nearly dilated—you're nearly done. This baby is ready to come out." Then she tore out of the room to find the doctor.

Since the doctor was busy with a C-section, I did some nice slow pushes for about an hour. No one yelled at me to push. Then the doctor came in. I did two or three hard pushes. At noon on November 21, 1990, out slipped Elizabeth Marie at 7 pounds, 13 ounces.

I was exhausted, but I was savoring how wonderful the birth had been and how beautiful my daughter was. My mom had gotten there shortly before Elizabeth's arrival. We were having this nice family moment. Until . . .

"You're going to have to push out the placenta," my doctor said.

I had been at this for twenty-four hours. I could barely speak, let alone move. Pushing seemed completely out of the question. "No way! I'm way too tired. I can't even think about pushing."

"You're going to have to."

"No!"

I wouldn't budge. I admit I'm not the nicest person after I give birth—I barely like myself. "No way. I just pushed out a baby, isn't that enough?"

We argued back and forth for a little while until I had this contraction. The doctor looked at me. *"Push!"*

"Okay. Okay." I squeezed my eyes shut and bore down.

When I opened them, all I could see was this red streak flying out of me. I blinked and looked at David. His eyes were bugged out and his mouth was hanging open like he'd just witnessed some amazing stunt. He was staring at the nurse, so I looked at her, too. My placenta was stuck to her face like a pie thrown by the Three Stooges. Her palms were open and her arms were stuck out at her sides. She was frozen and completely silent.

The wall behind the nurse—and several feet from me—was also splattered with blood. The hospital was being renovated and I remember thinking, "It's a good thing they haven't done the wallpaper yet."

The doctor cleared his throat and shook his head. "I've been doing this for a long time, and I've never seen anything like that before."

I couldn't speak. I was so tired and out of it. All I could think about was eating a large pizza and drinking an ice-cold Coke. Now that I remember it, I never did get them.

But my mother, dear mother of mine, put her hands on her hips and sort of growled at the doctor, "Well, you told her to push!"

The doctor looked at her sheepishly. Good old Mom. You can always count on your mother to come to your defense.

That birth taught me that I could do anything. Pushing that child out into the world is a feeling I can't describe. It's awe-inspiring. And that little trick with the placenta makes great cocktail-party conversation.

A WET BED AND NO BREAKFAST

Randi Bigelow, a mom and a doula from Needham, Massachusetts, thought she had time for a romantic weekend.

Everyone always says the first one's going to be late, so David and I thought we had nothing to worry about when we planned a romantic getaway in my thirty-eighth week. And why not? We needed one last fling before we became responsible adults.

We stayed at this quaint bed-and-breakfast in a little town in New Hampshire. We spent the day hiking around the mountains. We even bowled. I have a video of me waddling down the lane, my ball heading straight for the gutter every time. And that night, we had our last hurrah. Well, I had just drifted into blissful sleep when my water broke. It just drenched everything, the sheets, the mattress, the beautiful antique bed. I was frantically trying to wake up David, which is next to impossible because he's such a deep sleeper. I kept saying over and over, "My water broke. My water broke." Eventually, he drowsily asked, "What does that mean?"

"It means we have to leave."

Before we left, I tidied the place up a bit. Water was pouring out of me as I was fluffing the pillows and putting towels on the mattress. But it was useless; we had completely trashed the bed. We left the couple who owned the house a hastily scribbled note. *Sorry about the mess. Here's some extra money.*

During the ride back to Boston, my contractions were far enough apart that I knew I didn't have to worry. I turned the radio on and reclined in the seat. Closing my eyes, I said to David, "I don't care what you do. Just don't drive fast."

Well, he didn't drive fast, but he ended up lost. We stopped at the side of the road and it was pitch black outside. After what seemed like forever, a state trooper pulled up next to us. We told him I was in labor and we didn't know where we were. I just assumed he'd escort us to the highway. Isn't that what they do in the movies? But he just pointed a few times. Soon we were on Route 95, heading toward Boston.

My contractions were a minute and a half apart, so I assumed we had time to stop at home and throw some things in a suitcase. I must have been further along than I thought because I was suddenly so confused. That's what happens when a woman's reaching her final stages of labor. I ended up packing ten pairs of socks and a ponytail holder.

I could barely walk to the car. I squatted every five feet. I couldn't sit down, so I leaned over backward on the front seat with my butt on the dashboard. Thankfully, the hospital was only a ten-minute drive away. Forty-five minutes after we raced to the hospital and three hours after my water broke on October 30, 1994, Adam was born, weighing in at 7 pounds, 6 ounces.

A few days later, David found the bed-and-breakfast key in his jacket. So we sent it with a note. *Sorry about the mess. We had a baby boy.* They sent us a congratulations card. We always wondered if they set a policy against booking women in such an advanced stage of pregnancy. We've also been tempted to show up and demand the breakfast we missed. But I think I'd rather just hide from that couple for the rest of my life.

HEY, DOES YOUR BIRD FLY?

Nancy, a doula from Ottawa, Canada, thought a naturist enjoyed bird watching. She had no idea what she'd really be looking at.

As a doula, I offer support to moms and dads having babies. I'm there from the moment labor begins until the baby's born. A few months before a birth, I go to the parents' home and interview them. During the conversation, I always ask if there's anything I ought to know that might have a bearing on the childbirth. This one time, a couple looked at me rather sheepishly. When this happens I brace myself for the worst–abuse, disease, you name it.

After a few uncomfortable seconds, the wife chirped, "We're naturists."

Relief washed over me, but I didn't understand why she seemed so embarrassed. I'm also wondering, What the hell does bird watching have to do with childbirth? But sometimes people just like to talk.

Although I'm not an avid bird watcher, I love looking at them. I imagined we'd have conversations about various avian species. I thought maybe the mom would enjoy focusing on the birds fluttering by the window during her labor. In the process, maybe I'd learn a thing or two about our winged friends. I always like to expand my knowledge.

"That's really neat," I said.

They looked at each other and smiled, as if a great burden had been lifted. "We like to be open about it."

"Well, I'm glad you told me," I said. "I like to know as much as possible about my clients."

We talked a few times before the due date. I'd ask questions about the mom's appetite and health. Occasionally, I'd try to weave in birds. I figured it would make them feel more comfortable with me.

"Oh, you'll appreciate this. There's a beautiful blue jay sitting on my lawn chair outside. Its coat is such a deep royal blue. It seems to be looking for bugs or worms."

"Huh? Oh . . . that's nice."

I brought up birds a few other times, but the mom always seemed indifferent. I began to suspect it was the husband who forced the bird watching and she wanted no part of it. Maybe that's why it was such an issue during the interview.

Their day finally came. I received a call from the dad that labor had begun. They wanted me to come to their house until it progressed to the point that they'd need to get to the hospital. That's my job. While the doctor and nurse have to tend to the more medical needs, I'm there with a facecloth, a massage and encouraging words. I threw a book on birds in my bag, just in case.

Driving to the house, I thought what a beautiful day it was even though it was bitter cold and it might be difficult to see any birds. I was glad I had packed my book.

I parked the car and rang the doorbell. The husband poked his head out, stood behind the door and slammed it shut as soon as I walked in. I figured he didn't want one of his cats to sneak outside on such a chilly day.

"How are you doing?" he said. That's when I noticed he was naked. Totally naked. I was looking at his penis. All I could think was, I'm staring right at this guy's wanker and I can't stop staring.

That's when it hit me. A *naturalist* is a bird watcher. A *naturist* is a naked man with his wanker dangling in front of me! Everything suddenly became crystal clear. No wonder they have towels on all their furniture! No wonder their walls were empty the first time I was here—they take their photos down when prudes like me come to visit. Today, though, the photos were up. They had thought I understood! I glanced at a picture of a couple standing on a rock looking at a waterfall with their naked butts right in my face.

I tried not to focus.

"It's getting really cold out there, isn't it?" I spoke, staring at my shoes. Then I went upstairs to the bathroom to help Debbie. I could deal with naked women. That's my job. It's those wankers that are hard to take. But when I went downstairs, there it was again, staring at me from a chair in the living room. The dad sat there with his legs wide open. He seemed quite proud of it.

"Hmmm, do you want to watch *Oprah*?" I suggested, my eyes practically burning a hole in the television.

For the next few hours I became really adept at making sure Mr. Wanker had his clothes on for one reason or another. Even though it was freezing, we all took walks outside—fully clothed in jackets, hats and scarves. I also discovered that naturists ate with their clothes on, so I was constantly making sure there was food. I'd say, "Pete, you have a lot of hard work ahead of you. You better eat something." He'd say, "But you just made me eat something a few minutes ago." I'd say, "Eat again. You have no idea how much food you need and you won't get anything at the hospital."

Finally, the mom was ready to give birth, so we—completely clothed—drove to the hospital. When we got there, the mom immediately took her outfit off, but the dad left his on. Since their doctor was not on call, the attending physician tried to compensate by telling me, "Let them have carte blanche. Anything they want."

I begged, "Oh no, don't tell them that. Please don't tell them that."

Anyway, they had a little girl. I don't know if she's a naturist. But every time anyone asks me if I like to watch the birds out of my dining room window, I always laugh. Yes, I guess I'm a bit of a *naturalist*, I say.

TRICK OR TREAT

Dave Maciolek, a writer from Neptune, New Jersey, tells how he blended a paint job, football, Halloween and the birth of his first son, Derek.

*M*y wife, Louisa, is a world-class nester. She had a laundry list of ways for me to feather our nest. These were not "ifs" or "maybes"—they had to be done pre-baby. I'd been pretty successful at accomplishing all my assigned tasks but had stalled on getting the living room painted. Was it laziness? Nah, but knowing that newborns have a range of vision of about ten inches, I wasn't too worried about my hour-old kid pointing out cracks or chips from his bassinet. Of course, Louisa had other ideas.

Saturday night rolls around and I've run out of excuses not to play Benjamin Moore, so I drag out the rollers, brushes, ladder and all the sundry crap for a paint job, and begin. By midnight, I'm so bored. I'm thinking about switching to Krylon and replicating subway graffiti on the ceiling.

Solution: beer. By three-thirty or four in the morning, I'm not bored, just loaded. So I stagger to bed. About two hours later, Louisa wakes me up and announces she's having contractions. So I'm now in the mental netherworld of intoxication, hangover and sleep-deprivation. I suppose the paint fumes played a part as well.

Luckily, the contractions were very, very far apart, and we didn't have to head for the hospital until three in the afternoon. By then I was sober but still tired and hungover.

So we head for the hospital. They check Louisa in and get her into bed. I'm rubbing her back. After an hour or two of this, I start feeling better—at least well enough to notice that in the delivery room they have a television. So I click it on and behold, it's the Giants playing the Redskins—a terrific rivalry—I think it was the last year the Giants won the Super Bowl.

Somewhere around halftime, they gave Louisa an epidural. Perfect timing! So while all that nonsense took place on the screen, I focused my undivided attention on my wife.

The epidural slowed the process down a bit. The contractions were about three minutes apart, and every time she'd have one, I'd have to stand up, hold her hand, rub her back and take my eyes off the football game. After about a half hour of that, I was getting pretty tired of up-down, up-down all while trying to visualize the action I heard described on the gridiron.

Then I thought, "You pathetic wretch. You're complaining about a few knee bends and your wife is trying to pass a watermelon." Of course, those thoughts left my head as soon as the next point was scored.

The game ended, then there were no distractions, just contractions. I feared channel surfing might turn Louisa's mind toward thoughts of divorce, so I behaved myself.

By the time Derek was born, I guess I was kind of slap-happy. I saw the placenta, and I asked the doctor if he'd put it between a couple of slices of rye for me.

Mother and child—big child, he was 8 pounds, 12 ounces—settled into a room. I headed home, desperate for something to eat (the doctor had ignored my request) and a few hours' sleep.

But I was to pay for my sins. It was now Halloween, and my idiot neighbor had toilet-papered my other car, both trees on the front lawn, and so "mummified" my house that I had to hack my way past the front door with shears from the garage.

I looked at my living room paint job. The walls didn't quite match. The paint had been from two different batches. There'd be more penance for that, too.

HERE'S YOUR KEEPSAKE TUMOR
AND PLACENTA, MRS. PEETE

Actress Holly Robinson Peete and husband, Rodney Peete, quarterback for the Washington Redskins, were doubly thrilled to discover they were going to be parents—of twins. Holly, who got her first break on *21 Jumpstreet* and then went on to star in *Hangin' With Mr. Cooper* and *For Your Love,* has this vivid memory of childbirth.

I am probably the only person in the world who couldn't wait to have a C-section. I had carried these two acrobats in my stomach for all these months. They were doing back flips right and left and kicking every organ in reach. It was pretty painful.

To make matters worse, I had this fibroid tumor that was on the outside of my uterus. It was harmless but huge—about the size of a grapefruit. I felt like I was carrying triplets. There was no room left. The tumor stuck out on the left side of my stomach. People would come up to me and put their hands on me and say, "Isn't that cute? I can feel the baby's head." I'd go, "Uh-uh, honey. It isn't cute. It's the demon within."

The doctor said I could try it naturally, but I might be in labor for a long time. I figured with twins I didn't want any guesswork or worrying—I opted for a C-section. We planned it for October 17, 1997—a day Rodney wouldn't be away playing football.

I got to the hospital early in the morning. I'm a blood-and-guts kind of chick, so I planned to watch everything. After my epidural—which, I must say, was fabulous—the anesthesiologist put up a mirror for me because I really wanted to look at the babies being pulled out. It was an image I wanted to have with me for the rest of my life. I needed to see the actual moment when my babies touched the air. Rodney's not squeamish either—we're blood-and-guts soul mates. He was comforting me while the doctors were cutting me up, but he also kept glancing down to see what was going on. He didn't want to miss seeing my insides.

At one point, I even asked one of the surgeons to step back a little so I could have a better angle. He just laughed and scooted out of the way. He looked at me like I was insane. I said, "I'm sorry. I just want to see what you're doing. I don't know how many times I'll be able to be in here to watch you do this. This may be the last time for me."

Rodney Jackson came out first weighing 6 pounds, 1 ounce. Two minutes later, Ryan Elizabeth was pulled out weighing 4 pounds, 13 ounces. When he gets older, I'm sure RJ will try to work that two-minute age difference. He'll think he can boss his sister around because he's so much older.

Seconds after they came out, they were weighed and cleaned up. I know this will sound crazy, but as I watched them, I thought I saw my baby son wink at me. It was like he was saying, "Hey, Mama. I know who you are." I stared at the two of them for the longest time. It looked to me like they grabbed hands and snuggled next to each other. Mind you, my perception was a little blurred, but the nurses told me that this often happens with twins because they've been so close together for so many months. They don't want any space between them.

Then it was time to deal with the enemy. I wanted to watch as they lopped that horrible monster of a tumor off. They said they could sew me back and let it shrink down as my pregnancy hormones diminished, but I wanted that thing out of me more than I wanted the babies out. It was the demon. So the doctors cut it out.

The doctors thought I was crazy when I said, "I want to look at that thing face-to-face," but they were accommodating. A doctor put it in a jar of formaldehyde. He said, "Okay. Take this. You can look at it all you want." I had it in my room at the hospital. I admit it was kind of gross. I know everyone in that hospital thought I was mad, but as I said, I'm a blood-and-guts kind of girl.

My husband, on the other hand, was obsessed with the placentas. So they put the two placentas in another container for us. Rodney was so fascinated by them.

We had a full-on science lab in that hospital room. We had the two placentas and the tumor. We really disgusted some of our visitors. I'd say to them, "Do you want to see the tumor, the placentas or the babies?" They just looked at me like maybe this pregnancy thing had made me completely lose my mind.

6

Macho, Macho Men

The bigger they come, the harder they fall, puke, faint . . .

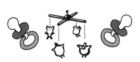

SO . . . HOW DOES THAT NEW CARPETING LOOK?

Lauren Annunziata of White Plains, New York, found that you don't really need painkillers when you're too busy worrying about your clumsy hubby.

$\mathcal{M}$y water broke at seven in the morning. At the time, I didn't know my water broke—it was five weeks too early. I just figured this was another weird by-product of my pregnancy. At two in the afternoon, I was on the phone with a friend and I mentioned it. She said, "Heelllllllo! Your water broke!"

I said, "I can't have the baby now. I'm having carpeting laid in the house. The carpet guy is here!"

Despite the carpet guy, I went to my doctor, who told me I needed to be admitted to the hospital. This baby was on its way. I called John, my husband, and he met me there. It was 4 P.M.

My house wasn't the only place being renovated; so was the hospital. It was jammed with people, and because of the construction, there wasn't enough room for everyone. Women were giving birth out in the halls, where the gurneys were lined up like box-cars. Luckily, we'd arranged in advance for a private room, where I was soon hooked up to a fetal monitor. All night I listened to my baby's heartbeat—when it wasn't drowned out by the screams of women giving birth out in the halls. When I'd hear a new baby cry, though, I'd feel a tinge of jealousy.

At two in the morning, they decided to move me. The nurse wanted to get me into a rocking chair to see if that would help my labor progress. Well, it's all a big blur to me without my glasses. I'm being lifted, but through the fog I see what looks like my husband falling to the floor. Then I hear a crash. Everyone lets go of me to run over to my husband. I plop into the rocking chair.

I'm squinting to decipher the chaos. All I can determine is that there's a bunch of people huddled on the floor by my husband. "Oh my God, what's wrong?" I shout to the crowd.

Nobody answers, and I'm attached to a monitor so I can't move. I'm screaming, "My husband! My husband!"

John can't stand hospitals. He hates them more than anyone I know. There hadn't even been any blood yet, but he had passed out, banging his nose on the way to the floor. His nose had hit the dresser drawer handle so hard, the knob broke off! Blood was everywhere. Even with my feeble eyesight, I could see his blood.

Now I've nearly forgotten I'm in labor. They get him up off the floor. He's all wobbly. They tell him he has to go to the emergency room, but he doesn't want to have anything to do with the emergency room. He's pleading with them to let him stay with me, but they're adamant. He's got to get his nose looked at, they say. It could be broken.

Suddenly he's gone. According to the fetal monitor, I'm having serious contractions. But I was so worried about John, I barely noticed them.

He was in the emergency room for close to three hours. When he came back, his nose was bandaged. Then my contractions started feeling a lot worse.

At 8 A.M. I was still only five centimeters dilated. The nurse suggested John take a shower. He looked at me. "Don't worry about your wife. She's nowhere near ready. We're going to be here for a while," the nurse assured us. John went into the shower in our room. Then the doctor walked into the room. He checked me and goes, "Okay, let's get her going now. She's ready."

Somehow John heard this and burst back into the room. He was dripping wet, holding a skimpy towel around his waist.

"Wait for me!"

We all laughed at poor John with the bandage on his nose and the tiny towel around his waist. My husband is in worse shape than I am.

"You can dry off," the doctor said. "We still have a little time."

Despite, or perhaps because of, all this pandemonium, the birth was really easy. I pushed a little and out popped Jason at a quarter to ten on May 18, 1995. He was 6 pounds, 1 ounce. Because he was born five weeks early, they put him in intensive care. I was bleeding a little, so the doctor told me I had to lie perfectly flat. John kissed me and went home to check on our daughter and get the house ready for our arrival.

So I'm relaxing blissfully when the fire alarm goes off. At first I think, False alarm. Then I see people racing past my room. They're evacuating my wing! I can't reach the call button. I was on so many drugs, I knew if I stood up I would have passed out. At first I thought, Oh, they know I'm here. But a few minutes went by and no one came for me. People ran back and forth. It seemed like hours. Then it got quiet. I imagined I'd go up in smoke. I was so high from the epidural, the idea of burning didn't seem entirely unpleasant.

Finally someone poked a head in the room. "Oh my God, we forgot all about you."

"Yeah, well, here I am," I said.

It turned out something had exploded outside by a construction site and caused a little fire. My wing of the hospital had lost power. So now they had to move me from my private room to a shared one. I was worried about Jason; I needed to see him. Once they showed my beautiful little baby to me, I felt much better.

I was released, but Jason had to stay in the hospital for two nights. I was crying hysterically because I didn't want to leave my little newborn son in the hospital. On Sunday, the doctors called us at about eight in the morning and said we could pick him up. I said, "Okay. We'll be right there." Then I shut my eyes.

At eleven, the phone woke us up. "Mrs. Annunziata, don't you want to pick up your son?" I felt so guilty. When we got to the hospital the poor little guy was starving, and I had to nurse him in a storage closet because there was no room anywhere else.

John likes to say that that was the worst night of his life. The next day, he bumped into some friends. Seeing his nose, they joked, "What did you do? Pass out in the delivery room?" He laughed and said, "As a matter of fact, I did." But I don't think they believed him.

I tell my friends that John's injury was better than any epidural. I completely forgot about my pain. I put so much energy into worrying about John that the contractions seemed to magically disappear until he returned. Maybe that's what men have to do—break their noses to distract their wives.

THE MAN WHO PIDDLED HIMSELF AND OTHER STORIES

Cindy Kerbs from West Columbia, South Carolina, has been a labor nurse for eighteen years. She's seen it all and then some.

I really hate to sound down on men, but they just give me so much ammunition. The biggest laughs I've had as a labor nurse always seem to be at the expense of men. These daddies get so nervous. Here are my favorite moments:

AND SHE TRUSTED HIM WITH SCISSORS?

We give the daddies official outfits. They're scrub clothes just like the doctors wear. This one daddy's dressed in his scrubs, holding his wife's hand, when he runs out to go to the bathroom. Well, he's gone for the longest time. We're waiting and waiting. I'm thinking that maybe he's sick in the bathroom.

I go to the nurses' station to check on some things when the daddy comes over to me. He's got a plastic bag in front of his pants. He looks at me real sheepishly and goes, "I need another pair of pants." I say, "What do you mean? Those pants look fine." He looks down as he says softly, "I piddled in my pants."

Me, being the consummate professional, exclaim, *"You what?"*

It turns out the poor guy had tied such a tight knot in his scrubs that he couldn't undo it when he went into the bathroom, and he really had to go. After many attempts, the urge was too great and he let go, right in his pants.

In this business people are always catching you off guard like that, but I recover as fast as I could and say, "Oh, these things happen. It's not a problem." I hand him another pair of pants and a scissor with a straight face. But the minute he walks out, the whole nurses' station erupts into laughter. We're falling on the floor with cramps. I hope he didn't hear us.

The birth went great. After his son was born, the guy was able to laugh about it. But I still cringe when I think about how hard it must have been for this guy to tell me he had wet his pants.

SAY, WHILE YOU'RE DOWN THERE, WILL YOU LOOK FOR MY CONTACTS?

This father came into the delivery room very enthusiastic. He was in charge—the coach. He had everything under control. "This is going to be great," he said, clapping his hands as if he had just given the plays for a football game.

And he's there for his wife. He's supportive. He's encouraging. "What can I do for you, honey?" he asks. He wipes her forehead. He rubs her back. He whispers encouragement.

This was a natural birth and at around five centimeters it gets pretty intense. The contractions were very strong and this woman was in a lot of pain. She's doing fine, but she's screaming.

The next thing I know, the husband's disappeared from her side. I look around the room and he's curled up in the fetal position in a La-Z-Boy. He's not watching. He's not moving. He's rolled into a ball in his own world.

When the baby finally emerges, the guy doesn't even notice. He's still curled up. But his wife is determined to have him participate in the birth. She's telling him to come over and cut the cord. She keeps calling him.

At first the guy doesn't move. But I think he was just so embarrassed by his uselessness that he decided to redeem himself, and he cut the umbilical cord. He crawls from the La-Z-Boy to the birthing chair. He's still on his hands and knees as he cuts the cord. Actually, he's practically lying on the floor because he can't do any more than that. He's just so outdone and overwhelmed.

He cuts the cord and then crawls back to the La-Z-Boy and gets right back into the fetal position. His wife, the doctor and I are going, "What in the world?"

I don't really know what happened. There wasn't any blood. Sure, there was pain. But I honestly believe it all of a sudden hit him that he was no longer in control. Most men want to be the rescuer, the savior, the hero. In childbirth, that isn't the case. The woman's body just does what it's going to do.

WERE THOSE MATTE OR GLOSSY?

I'm helping this woman as she's in the final stages of pushing. She's had an epidural, so she's not in excruciating pain. Actually, it's quite manageable. As she's pushing, from the corner of my eye I see her husband fumbling with a camera. He's pressing the wrong buttons and dropping the camera. In between pushes, his wife's telling him what to do.

"Hit the button on the top. No, not that one. The one next to it. No!" She's yelling at him, but he's fumbling. He's sweating. He's shaking.

Finally she just reaches across me toward him. As I'm watching, I'm amazed by how long her arms suddenly seem. It's like these six-foot arms are stretching out for the camera. "Give me that camera," she says, completely frustrated by her husband. She grabs it and reels it in toward her.

She's pushing and pushing and finally the baby's head starts peeking out. She sits upright and starts snapping away as the baby's coming out of her. Her husband's watching with his mouth hanging open. I swear, sometimes women are superhuman.

SORRY, WRONG WOMB

This woman was being prepped for an emergency C-section. I told her husband, who looked pretty dazed, to go to her room and wait for the surgery to begin. He headed down the hall, walked into a room and held the woman's hand. He's stroking her hand and whispering to her, "It's going to be okay." Then he looks up. There's another man across the bed from him just staring at him. He looks down again and realizes this is not his wife! He's in the wrong room. "Sorry," he says. I found him and walked him back to his wife's room.

AS A MATTER OF FACT, I LOOK EXACTLY LIKE THAT DOWN THERE!

This couple wanted the sex of the baby to be a surprise. So the doctor tells the husband, "When the baby comes out, I'm going to let you tell us its sex."

So the baby's born and the doctor's holding the baby's bottom up. The daddy gets all excited. "It's a boy! It's a boy!" The doctor, the nurses and I are all looking at one another. There's no doubt about it—it's a girl. Finally, the doctor goes, "You better go into the bathroom and have another look at yours, because this is a girl."

I don't know what he thought he saw, but these daddies just don't think or see like we think or see. That's for sure.

GOODFELLA MAKES GREAT DAD

Even though actor Ray Liotta often plays menacing psychos, he's really a softy—especially when it came to the birth of his daughter, Karsen.

It was about 11:00 A.M. when the doctor induced my wife, Michelle. They said our baby would be born around 6 or 7 P.M. But at 1 P.M. things started speeding up. I knew it would be any minute. Suddenly there was all this excitement in the room.

I don't think I've ever been so thrilled in my life. I was adopted and always felt like I never really had a history. So for me, this baby was the beginning of a family tree. I was standing next to Michelle, holding one of her legs, and suddenly it was all too much. I started feeling really, really light-headed. Whoa, I'm getting emotional just talking about it right now! It's funny how that stuff just comes up. Anyway, I had to sit down or I would have passed out.

We knew we were having a girl. We wanted to know the sex because there's a whole lot of shopping to be done. We started picking out a name early on. My wife didn't like typical girls' names. She had come up with some really bizarre names like Ming. We both liked the name Sydney, but one of our four dogs already had that tag. Finally, we both agreed on Karsen.

We both were really into the whole "talking to the belly" thing. I'd say, "Hey, Karsen, what's going on? I'm Daddy. I can't wait to meet you."

When Karsen was born, she came out crying hysterically. She wouldn't stop. She was worked up in this frenzy. So I reached over and said, "It's okay, Karsen. Relax. It's Daddy." I put my hand on her and she just stopped cold. She knew her name and the sound of my voice. I was tearing up because it was all so emotional for me.

Before Karsen was born I had taken a tour of the hospital and noticed all these surveillance cameras by the doors. I asked why there were cameras everywhere and was told, "That's to make sure nobody steals the babies." Well, when I heard that I freaked out. "Steal the babies? Are you nuts?" So once Karsen was born, I never let her out of my sight.

When the nurses washed her up—boom—I was there. I stayed next to Karsen when they did the weigh-in and footprint. I memorized everything about her because I didn't want any switching. They nurses told me to go home to sleep, but I wouldn't leave. I was paranoid and I think a lot of it had to do with being adopted. Karsen never left my side.

After a few more hours of this, I just said, "We're out of here." Poor Michelle, I probably should have let her stay another night because she was so exhausted, but we went home. I remember thinking, "I'm taking my family home." I was starting my family tree.

HE DROPPED AND GAVE ME . . . NONE

Dr. Norman Armstrong of Falls Church, Virginia, has been an obstetrician for twenty-five years. After thousands of deliveries, this one stands out in his mind.

I've never had a dad drive me as nuts as Eric.

The guy was a graduate of the United States Naval Academy. I don't know if he was a typical graduate, but he was very, very rigid. He'd accompany his wife to appointments. He'd even make appointments for his wife. If I said, "I'll see you next week at four," he'd reply, "We'll see you at sixteen hundred hours." I almost saluted.

He'd try to order me around. He'd say, "We had an appointment at fourteen hundred. Why are you late?"

I sat him down and explained. "You know, a 2:00 appointment is really great. And I could meet all my appointments if I didn't have to talk to anybody. If I just did what I needed to and let you go, that's no problem. Two o'clock would be easy. But invariably you or your wife have some questions and you multiply that by so many people during the day, that adds minutes and minutes to each visit. After a while, 2:00 is no longer 2:00."

After that, we understood each other. But it was a standoff. There was definitely some tension in the air.

His wife, Beth, didn't make any decisions or ask any questions. Everything had to be approved by Eric. He questioned and decided. I'd ask her how she felt. He'd say, "Fine." One day, I had enough. I said, "I do believe she's the patient." His response? "Yes, but I'm paying the bills."

So the day of the delivery arrived and in walked Eric in his dress whites. We needed sunglasses for the reflections off his brass. I couldn't believe it. I nearly laughed in his face. But he was very serious. He came into that delivery room like he owned it. He expected everything to be perfect and shipshape.

He wanted to know how long the labor would last. He couldn't understand why I didn't have a precise answer. He helped his wife with breathing and counting, but he couldn't comprehend why there was no rhyme or reason to her pain. I think he expected the contractions to follow orders.

I think he allowed his wife to have an epidural because it was a way to control the contractions. They were like sailors who wouldn't follow orders. They needed to be court-martialed.

So finally the head came out. We delivered the baby and clamped the cord. I turned to show Eric his daughter, and the guy's eyes rolled to the back of his head and he passed out flat on his face. Most people faint and their arms and legs are askew, but Eric fell perfectly, like a plank, with military posture. It was hilarious. I nearly peed in my pants.

Once we figured out he was breathing, we left him alone. He had been such a pain in the neck that nobody wanted to revive him. Even his wife was laughing. It never occurred to any of us that he could have broken his nose. The nurses said, "Should we do something?" I said, "Let's just leave him alone."

I imagine he's had other children since then, but I didn't

deliver them. I doubt I met his requirements for a physician. He needed somebody who was very, very serious. I think I'm appropriately serious, but I joke around, too. Deliveries should have a little levity to them, as long as everything's going well. He didn't share my sense of humor.

I always say the minute this job stops being fun, I'll give it up. Thankfully, I haven't run into too many Erics to make me do just that.

DID HE HAVE MATCHING SCRAPPY DOO SOCKS?

Suzi Coleman, a doula from Phoenix, Arizona, witnessed this bizarre act.

I helped deliver the baby of a woman who was so modest she wore her bra underneath the hospital gown. Most women whip everything off to get comfortable. They don't care if their butt's sticking in the air. They just want to get the baby out.

Her husband was very concerned that this might never happen. He looked at me and said, "She is the most modest person I know."

She was stuck at five centimeters for the longest time. We wanted to get her into the shower because hydrotherapy can help move labor along. But of course she'd have to get naked. I mentioned this to her husband.

"She'll never do it," he said. "Never. I know my wife. She won't get naked in front of all these people." Besides her husband and me, there was a nurse and a doctor in the room.

"These people have seen plenty of naked women," I said.

"It doesn't matter. My wife barely lets me see her naked," he joked.

As he was testifying to his wife's modesty, I saw a flurry of activity out of the corner of my eye. His wife was stripping. She couldn't get out of her clothes fast enough.

"As I said, we're going to have to figure something out because my wife is just too modest."

His modest wife was standing in the middle of the room naked. I nodded to her husband. "Hey, I don't think we have a problem here."

He looked shocked.

As I started helping his wife into the bathroom, I saw another flurry of activity from the corner of my eye. Now it's the husband's turn to peel. I saw the shirt and the pants come off. I've heard stories about husbands who get completely naked with their wives, so I squeezed my eyes shut.

When I opened them, the husband had stripped only as far as his Scooby Doo boxers. We laughed and laughed over those Scooby Doo boxers. Then he got into the bathtub with his wife. He rubbed her and held the shower nozzle against her back. They were in the bath for an hour and a half. The baby was born three hours later. No, it wasn't named Scooby.

THE GREEN GIANT

Melinda, a personal trainer from the Los Angeles area, has a cautionary tale for women married to big, macho guys.

I've been a personal trainer for ten years, and my husband, Jeff, is quite an athlete himself. He was a lineman on his college football team, worked at night as a bouncer, has a black belt in kung fu, and, if that isn't enough, he's a little over six-five and weighs in at a very muscular two-fifty. Pretty imposing, right? Well, my big, tough husband was knocked cold by a 7-pound baby.

Being very health conscious, we both took my pregnancy very, very seriously. I read everything I could get my hands on, from domestic books on nutrition for expectant mothers to their Asian counterparts, which have some interesting viewpoints. Anyway, by the time my due date rolled around, I felt incredibly excited and pretty confident.

We both had attended the birthing classes. I thought Jeff looked a little squeamish when they showed those gory videos, but I wasn't sure—the lights were dim. Then I thought to myself, Nah. Jeff broke a couple of ribs and some fingers playing ball. I'd attended to his broken nose after a kung fu sparring. He didn't seem to give it much more thought than a hangnail.

When I went into labor, we were both very calm. We had rehearsed everything. I grabbed my bag. We called the doctor. He said to come right in, and so on. First we spent about an hour or two in the triage room. Then, when I was at four centimeters, they moved me into the delivery room. Although I wanted to do it naturally, the pain was intense and I wasn't about to be a hero. I asked for an epidural. When the anesthesiologist wheeled in his tray and started getting my back ready, that's when things changed.

You know how people talk about somebody being seasick or nauseated and turning green? I always thought that was a figure of speech. It's not. I was talking to Jeff as the doctor gave me the epidural. First, his face just kind of fell, like the muscles in it turned to soup or something. Then he turned green. I mean green—green like grass, green like moss, green like I've never ever seen on a human being before or since. Then he clapped a hand to his mouth and his cheeks puffed out.

"Not on me," I yelled at him.

I guess I must have jerked as I said that, because behind me the anesthesiologist yelled, "Stay still!"

I turned my head to answer him, and he shouted, "Sit down! Sit down!" I was already sitting on the bed, and I was thinking, This guy has lost his mind. He's yelling at me to sit down, I am sitting down, and he's not even looking at me while he's yelling!

Then I heard the crash. The anesthesiologist was looking at and talking to Jeff. He could tell he was about to pass out, and he wanted him to sit down. But he couldn't turn away from his work on me.

"Oh my God!" There's my giant flat out on the floor, in a puddle of his own vomit. I wanted to hop off the bed and help him, but by then the nurse was trying to rouse him. Pretty soon his eyes opened, but he just lay there. I was yelling to him, "Jeff! Jeff!" but he wasn't answering, and I was freaking out! The anesthesiologist finished up on me and ran over to help. The two of them could barely lift Jeff's head. The nurse ran out of the room and came back with two more nurses. The four of them got him sitting up. Then he looked at me and said, "Baby, are you all right?" They very slowly helped him into a chair, and he began turning from green back to his natural color.

A doctor examined him, and luckily, he hadn't hit his head on the way down. They checked his blood pressure and got him something to drink.

We just sat there for a few hours, riding the contractions and watching the little waves on the monitor. Then it was time to push. I had about two hours of hard pushing, and finally, the baby began to crown. The doctor asked Jeff if he wanted to have a look, so he got up and came around between the stirrups. By now, I'm too busy to worry about Jeff, but thank God, one of the labor nurses was watching him. Suddenly, she grabbed him by the arm and pulled him back into the chair. He fainted again, dead away.

Little Connor was born weighing just over 7 pounds, and big daddy missed it.

7

Surprise!

A good scout tries to "be prepared."
But it's the baby who calls the shots.

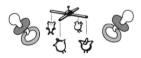

KNOCKED OUT

It took the author's mom, Catherine Zutell, a fastball to the skull to convince her that she was pregnant.

I didn't know I was pregnant for the first three months. Your father and I had been married for six years and we wanted babies from the start. We were beginning to think something was wrong. And then I finally thought I might be expecting, but I didn't want to get my hopes up. I found out I had an aunt who went through the change of life when she was barely thirty. I thought, Maybe that's what's happening to me. I know this all makes me sound really ditzy.

In those days there were no over-the-counter pregnancy tests. You brought your urine to the pharmacy and they analyzed it. I finally got the nerve and called the drugstore, but the pharmacist needed to give the report to my doctor. Well, my doctor had died years earlier and I'd never found another one. As you know, I'm the world's biggest procrastinator. And so another month goes by. And then another.

It was a beautiful Saturday afternoon in May when your father and I went on a picnic with some friends. We were playing softball. I have no idea what my position was. I think I was standing on one of the bases watching the clouds. Your father threw the ball at me, but I wasn't paying attention. I must have turned because the ball whacked me on the back of the head and I passed out. I was unconscious for a few seconds. When I came to, everyone suggested I go to a doctor.

Of course I procrastinated. But a few days later Aunt Bernadette took me to her doctor. He grilled me on my medical history for his files. He asked if my periods were regular.

"Well, as a matter of fact, no," I said.

"Did you ever think you could be pregnant?"

"I want to be so much, but I'm so afraid of finding out I'm not. I just think something's wrong with me."

As I'm talking the doctor touches my stomach. "Your stomach feels like you are."

Then he gives me an internal exam. "You're about three months pregnant." I couldn't believe what the doctor was saying and I made him tell me again.

I was ecstatic. I loved every minute of being pregnant. I felt great. All my life I wanted to be a mother and it was finally happening. I couldn't wait for you to be born.

You were a week late and I got to a point where I didn't feel like I was ever going to really give birth. Your father's birthday is October 26, so I made him a special dinner of lamb chops. I set up a card table in the living room and lit candles. We ate the dinner, which was delicious. I cleared the dishes and lit the candles on the birthday cake.

I turned off the lights and began singing "Happy Birthday" while carrying the cake down the hall. All of a sudden, my water broke. It was a deluge. I was frozen. But your father was so calm. He blew out the candles, shut everything off and got my bags. Then we headed for the hospital. It was about 8 P.M.

Your father was so excited to have a child born on his birthday. You, however, had other plans. I was in labor for twelve hours.

Labor was terrible. They say you forget the pain, but I still remember. I didn't have any drugs. The doctor even sent Daddy home at about midnight. She told him to get some sleep and come back in the morning. That's what they did in those days. But at 4:30 A.M. you were born, weighing 7 pounds, 6 ounces.

I saw you right away. I can still see you–that scrunched-up face in the dark room with the lights shining down. You were so cute. That was the happiest day of my life. It was so beautiful. When your sister was born two years later, she looked exactly like you. That was my second happiest day. No, I better not say it like that. They were both the happiest days of my life.

The next summer we went to another picnic and the talk turned to my baseball injury. I suddenly realized that the doctor never did check the bump on my head. I think I'm all right, though.

NEXT STOP—BABY

After driving a Los Angeles bus for sixteen years, Evelyn Davis knew exactly what to expect—until she met a passenger who was expecting.

It was 7 A.M. and I had just gotten behind the wheel of my bus. I pulled out of the layover zone at Maple and Seventh and started my assignment, just like any other day. I stared out the window at another perfect Los Angeles morning.

I made a couple of stops. More and more people got on. I exchanged "Hellos" and "How are yous" with some of the regulars. When I got to Hill Street and Seventh, which is the third stop on my route, one of the passengers yelled, "There's a lady in labor!"

I turned around and looked. "What?" A woman pointed to the lady sitting beside her. I said, "How can she be in labor? She doesn't even look pregnant."

She was a small woman and I couldn't even see a belly on her.

But then I looked her in the eye and saw that this woman was in a whole lot of pain. She was gritting her teeth and squeezing her eyes while holding her stomach. Suddenly, a big wave of pain must have ripped through her because she bolted up in her seat.

The woman was now standing in front of her seat squeezing her legs together as if she could somehow keep this baby from coming out. This woman wasn't just in labor—this woman was about to give birth.

A few passengers grabbed her and tried to get her to lie down on the seats or the floor. At first she resisted. She was frozen there, holding her legs together. Somehow, they got her to stretch out on the floor, but they had her feet facing the windows. I said, "If she starts having this baby it will be born under the seats. We'll never be able to get to him." As they turned her around the long way, I phoned the dispatcher, telling them to get an ambulance to Hill Street right away.

There were about eight or nine passengers on the bus. So when I realized we weren't going anywhere, I issued some of them transfers so they could take another bus. I guess a lady having a baby on their bus wasn't a good enough excuse for being late to work. Almost everyone got off except two ladies. I don't think any of us realized that we'd actually be delivering this baby. We believed the paramedics would get there in time and save the day.

But when I turned around, she'd taken her pants off. She was ready to go. One woman's rubbing her stomach. The other woman is Hispanic, just like Susana, the mom-to-be. The woman giving birth didn't speak a word of English and my Spanish is very limited. So the Hispanic woman translated everything Susana was saying.

We didn't really need words. We had a ton of eye contact. I felt like she understood everything I was trying to tell her. And in a strange way, I understood what she was saying, too. With my eyes, I told her to trust me. I told her I was there to help her and that she didn't have to worry. I told her I knew what I was doing—even though I had no idea what I was doing. I have a son and a daughter. My daughter was born cesarean. My son was born vaginally, but I had no idea what was going on down there.

I could tell by the way Susana looked at me that she trusted me. I could also see that this baby was almost here. I wasn't nervous—I was excited. I was a little bit in shock that something like this was happening on my shift. I'd been driving a bus for sixteen years, and it's pretty ordinary. People get on. People get off. People ask for transfers. People talk about the weather. No one has babies.

I ran up to the front of the bus to look out the side-view mirror for the paramedics. There was nothing behind us. Where were those guys? Hurry up, I silently pleaded. I stared at the mirror hoping I could will them to my bus. But nothing. When I looked back there was water gushing down the aisle. I knew Susana's water bags had burst. It was like a flood on the bus. I looked at the woman. The baby's head was crowning.

This is really going to happen. Right now. There's no time to be scared. There's no time to react. Women have been doing this all over the world without help from a doctor or a paramedic. We can do it, too.

I got on my knees. I held onto the baby's head and sort of turned it sideways so the little body would come through okay. I was going on instinct. The mother pushed and within seconds the baby was out. I rubbed its chest and prayed. I prayed and prayed for Mommy and Baby as I massaged its chest and little face. Suddenly out came *"Wwhhhhhhhhhhhhhhhhhhhhhhhhhaaaaaaaaaaaaaaaaaaaaa"* in the cutest, sweetest voice I'd ever heard. It was a little tinny whine, but it was a sound that let me know everything was going to be fine. I swear it was the best noise I'd ever heard. Then I placed Baby on Mommy's stomach. They stared at each other like they were saying hi.

When I looked up again there were the paramedics. They took over. And suddenly I was pushed out of the bus.

As I stood outside, I realized I didn't know whether the baby was a boy or a girl. I didn't even look there. I tried to get back on the bus, but they wouldn't let me. "We can handle it from here," they told me. I said, "All I want to know is, is it a boy or a girl?" They told me it was a boy. I had secretly wished it to be a girl so Susana could name it after me. I imagined her telling her daughter, "You're named after Evelyn, the bus driver, who delivered you." When I found out it was a boy, I thought Metro would be cute, but she named the 6-pound, 6-ounce baby Juan Jose.

In truth, I didn't have much to do with it anyway. I was basically the catcher. Little Juan Jose delivered himself. He was ready to come out on my bus. Maybe he liked the ride. For me, it was such a natural thing. I felt like I'd been doing it all my life. Now just thinking about it, I get all excited. I can see it like it happened today.

After the paramedics cleaned up, I took the bus back to the layover zone, washed my hands and went back on my route, just like any other day. I finished that portion of the day right on time. That night I went to the hospital with a little bouquet of flowers and a balloon. I kissed little Juan Jose's face. I gave his mommy a great big hug and said, "You may not understand this, but I am the godmother." She didn't know what I'd said, but she said something back to me in Spanish, which I didn't understand. Later someone translated it for me. "You'll always be his honorary godmother."

P.D.A. AND BIGHEADED BABIES

Kathy Campion, a labor nurse from Elk Grove, California, shared some of her more surreal delivery-room stories.

DID THEY PUT THE MIRROR ON THE CEILING?

There are times when you feel like an intruder in the delivery room. For instance, I once walked in on a naked woman in bed with her husband sitting behind her rubbing her nipples. Nipple stimulation releases hormones that cause contractions, so the husband thought he was being a big help.

A nurse friend also walked in on the same couple while Dad was massaging Mom's nipples. The mom was stretching her perineum, so she had her hands in her vagina. The nurse looked at them and goes, "Excuse me," and walked out. She said she felt like she was walking in on some sex act. Maybe she had!

BUT I NEED IRON!

Body piercing has gotten out of control. Not only is it amazing what people will pierce, but it's absolutely shocking to me that they'll keep the ring in place even as they near their delivery. They'll show up with rings in their labia and clitoris. I'm like, "It's time to let go. Would you rather have a baby or a ring?"

SHE NEVER WONDERED WHY HIS NICKNAME WAS "BLOCKHEAD"

I can't believe some of the things men will reveal to their wives while they're in labor. I remember this one woman was pushing out her baby. She was pretty uncomfortable, but she'd had an epidural. She asked me, "Does this baby have a big head or something?" And I said, "Yes, but it's moving along. You'll be okay." At that moment her husband pipes up and says, "I had the largest football helmet in high school. They had to get a specialist to make it for me."

The wife is in the middle of pushing, but she stops and looks at him. "You're telling me this now."

Well, she delivered quite a big baby, head and all. We put one of those little knit caps on him and it kept popping off his head.

A TRUE FALSE LABOR

Dana Streeter from Sherman Oaks, California, has been a labor and delivery nurse for ten years. She's seen the bizarre and then some. But her wildest childbirth story was the one that got away.

*W*e have a saying at the hospital: "The bus always unloads at five in the morning." For some reason, we just get inundated with moms around that time. We go, "The bus is here."

And they'll just roll in, one after another, until we're swamped with moms about to burst or moms who think they're about to burst.

And some of these moms are crazy. I'll tell you, women can get downright weird during labor. One of the stories that the nurses love to tell is about a woman who had orgasms throughout her delivery. It was a natural birth and she was moaning, "Ohhhh. Ohhh. OHHHHHH. This feels so good, Doctor. Ohhhh my God. Oh God. OH! . . ." And on and on. I know, I know. It's hard to believe anyone could feel that good in labor.

Then there are the women—usually on Demerol—who tell the doctor how wonderful their examination feels. They're going, "Oh, Doctor. Don't stop. Don't ever stop. Stay right there. Keep checking me."

It gets pretty embarrassing, but that's nothing compared to the cesarean-section moms. They get their drugs and are lying on the operating table—half in, half out of consciousness. Then, suddenly, they'll just grab the doctor's butt, or whatever appendage is within their reach. The doctor's yelling to the anesthesiologist, "Tie her down! Tie her down!"

There's no doubt that women get crazy. But these stories don't compare to my wildest encounter in the delivery room.

It was Christmas Eve three years ago when an ambulance pulled up and unloaded a pregnant woman on a gurney. As a nurse you figure, Okay. Who freaked out and called 911? It very rarely is a real emergency. When it comes to childbirth, people have a lot more time than they think.

I notice the woman is handcuffed to the bed. Next to her is a man—but this isn't her husband—it's a police officer. It turns out she'd been arrested for credit-card fraud and had gone into labor.

We uncuff her and she's pretty sick. It's coming out both ends. I'm asking her questions. She tells me she's seven months pregnant. I put on the monitor to check the baby's heart, but I'm not getting any heart tones. This concerns me, because the baby could be in fetal distress. I'm about to check her further but she gets sick again. Before I know it, she's jumped off the table and is back in the bathroom. From where I am, I can hear her heaving and heaving. It's horrible. I plead with her to come back out so I can give her some medicine and monitor the baby.

And then she's a blur out the door. I run down the hall and chase her. All I can see is her butt hanging out of the hospital gown. It turns out she wasn't pregnant at all, just fat and suffering from some food poisoning. She'd had a baby seven months before and was still very thick around the middle. She thought she had the perfect escape plan.

She made it off the hospital grounds, but security caught her a few blocks away. She was having an asthma attack. When they took her to the emergency room, I confronted her. "Why did you say you were pregnant?" She didn't answer me. She was so angry she'd been caught. She thought she could pull one over on the sympathetic nurses in labor and delivery.

LADEEES AND GENTLEMEN, CHILDREN OF AAALLLL AGES!

Dace Lavelle, a labor nurse at a hospital in Southern California, has been practicing her profession for over a decade. Having assisted in thousands of births, her memories run more toward a collection of snapshots than full-length stories.

One night a few years back, a woman came in with triplets. A rather rare occurrence, but what made it extra-special was that she was at thirty-seven weeks. Triplets usually are born quite a bit earlier (around thirty weeks), because it gets pretty crowded in there. A single baby at thirty weeks generally runs around three pounds. Twins, maybe two and a half, and triplets are usually only about two pounds each.

I was fortunate enough to "scrub the case," meaning I would assist the doctor with the cesarean. I handed the doctor the scalpel and within moments, to our total astonishment, he hands me a full-size baby—well over 6 pounds. A few moments later and he reaches in and pulls out another full-size baby! At this point, I don't know whether this reminds me more of the circus act where thirty-five midgets climb out of a Volkswagen or the magician pulling several fat rabbits out of his hat. The doctor dips his hands in again and comes up with . . . another full-size baby!

We were flabbergasted. Their combined weight was over twenty-one pounds. Then you have to figure in that for every five pounds of baby you have at least a pound of placenta. So that's another four-plus pounds. Then add in maybe six pounds of water and we're talking over thirty pounds of various stuff in this mommy's belly.

Speaking of the circus, I recently witnessed a feat of acrobatics worthy of Ringling Bros. A woman had been in labor for quite a while and the baby was just about ready to come out. The doctor was busy donning his gloves and asked the labor nurse to position a stool between the stirrups. She did but at the last moment noticed some water on the floor near the stool. Wanting to avert a slip, she moved the stool so she could mop up, but he was unaware. He sat down on empty space, hit the floor, rolled onto his back and, putting his hands on the floor, sprang back into a standing position. Without so much as taking a breath, he said, "Another pair of sterile six and a halves, please!" How's that for unflappable?

I remember one birth with a dad named Jose. He was incredibly excited about his wife's delivery—so much so that when the action got intense, he fainted. Well, somebody caught him on the way to the floor and gently laid him down. We cracked some salts under his nose, but it just wasn't bringing him around. Of course, this complicated things—because now we had to worry about Mom, the baby, seeing that the doctor was "covered" and an unconscious father lying on his back on the floor.

Not having the manpower to haul him down to emergency at that moment, I ran down the hall and grabbed a vital sign monitor and hooked him up. He was doing fine, but he just wouldn't come around. Pulse is fine, blood pressure okay, oxygenation fine.

The doctor was worried about him, and every minute or so he checked him, calling his name. "Jose! Jose, do you know where you are?" Jose's eyes would flutter but not quite focus. "I'm in your office," Jose would answer, never questioning why he was on a floor responding to someone standing over him. "Okay, go back to sleep," the doctor would tell him.

Well, we went through the same routine with the "Where are you?" question at least three or four times and got the same reply from Jose each time.

The last time it happened, Jose blinked fast, said, "Oh my God!" and jumped up like he was spring-loaded. We grabbed him by both arms and walked him to the scale for a look at his new baby boy. He grinned so wide we thought he'd crack his jaw.

DID YOU CONSIDER HAVING HER TRANSGENDERED?

Jan and Jim of Chicago have an interesting perspective on science, beliefs and planning.

*J*im and I have been married for ten years. I guess we should be the poster boy and girl for "likes attract." Because we're so alike, people sometimes think we're sister and brother instead of husband and wife. We're both really, really anal, as the Freudians like to say. If the fringe at the edge of a carpet is sideways, we straighten it out. We wear out a vacuum cleaner every two years or so—we're that kind of anal.

Once I became pregnant, we both had a whole new horizon of things to obsess over. After the sonogram, the doctor said it was a boy and we set about turning the spare bedroom into baby-boy heaven. We pored over catalogs from all kinds of furniture suppliers. Would we make it generic boy or a theme, and if so, which theme? There were Star Wars, Batman, Sesame Street, Nautical, Lodge, Safari, Western/Ranch, Desert, High Tech, LeMans, Alpine, Polynesian, Asian—it was insane!

We decided to decorate it in generic boy's-room style and as he matured, we would let him find the motif that reflected his choice of lifestyle. So blue was the order of the day. We went full bore, from a bassinet trimmed in robin's-egg blue to a crib bumper with navy accents. And, of course, it all had to be coordinated with the drapes, blinds, curtains, carpeting, wallpaper and trim paint. And what about his wardrobe? We found him a sailor suit and a navy blue blazer with khakis to match Daddy's.

We even searched far and wide for a photo album in just the right shade of sky blue to perfectly match the birth announcements. Our friends thought we were nuts, and we couldn't disagree, but it was just so much fun!

We never went through the same thing on names, because we had agreed right from the start that our son would be named after his daddy—James Jr.—making him James III, which had a pretty royal sound to it, right?

Well, finally my due date rolled around. I was being induced—no surprises, right? It was a cold day in February. We got to the hospital in exactly seventeen minutes (we'd rehearsed the drive like a dozen times). My bag had been packed weeks in advance, so I didn't have to worry about that. We had preregistered. Jimmy had a camera and a video camera. My mother and father arrived a few minutes after us. I delivered like the pizza man. Almost pain free, just a few pushes and voilà.

Then the doctor says, "Congratulations. It's a girl!"

I remember looking at Jimmy, who at that moment had the video camera up to his eye. He's looking right at my baby girl and says (and we have this on tape) to the doctor, "Are you sure?" The doctor laughs and holds the baby closer and says, "See for yourself." They put the baby on my chest, and I squint at its privates. No penis. So what. I didn't care. I was crazy about her.

We named her Jamie. We left the nursery paint job as it was. Jimmy and the men even smoked the IT's A BOY cigars they had bought months in advance. Pretty soon, our anally perfect house was a little sloppy. Not much, mind you, just a toy out of place or the carpet fringe a little crooked.

Jamie's almost three now, and she's messy as hell. And we love her like crazy. We're even trying to give her a brother or sister—we don't care which—and when I get pregnant, I'm not even going to find out the sex; we want to be surprised.

HEY, LADY, WHAT'S UNDER THAT SHEET?

Stel McGorrian, of Chicago, started her career as a nurse in a small hospital in Liberty, New York. One of her favorite births was a complete surprise.

I had been working at the hospital for only a few months and was very eager to make a good impression. Late one afternoon, a very large woman was brought in experiencing labor pains. She was at least 300 pounds and didn't seem to be the least bit nervous.

I checked her signs and she was a long way from delivering, so we kept her in the triage room, as was standard procedure. It was a small hospital and we all wore many hats, so I kept looking in on her every ten minutes or so, to be sure things weren't heating up.

Well, this went on for about an hour. The doctor, who was busy elsewhere, asked me how much she was dilated. With complete assurance, I told him, "She's only at two centimeters and her contractions are very far apart."

I continued my rounds, looking in on a couple of other patients, then looked at my watch and realized I was due back in triage to check on the woman. When I walked in she was giggling uncontrollably. Since there was nothing funny going on, I was very curious as to what had her tickled.

"What's so amusing?" I asked her.

"This!" she answered, as she pulled back the sheet and revealed a squirming infant on her abdomen.

I gasped with disbelief. She had been at two centimeters only ten minutes ago. At first I was amazed, and then terrified. I was certain my career at this hospital was over. I'd be branded incompetent and fired. As I racked my brain to think of how I would explain this to the doctor, he entered the room and saw the baby.

I looked at him with my mouth gaping and began to stammer. Before I could get a word past my lips, he laughed and said, "Don't worry, Nurse. This is Jenny. She always does that!"

I later learned that this woman had three older children who all were born with no more effort than a walk in the park.

IT'S NOT THE CHILI, IT'S THE CHILD

Bruce MacArthur, an executive from Darien, Connecticut, has two children, Chase and Elizabeth. As Bruce tells it, while neither baby arrived with any particular fanfare, it was hard to keep a straight face each time.

*B*efore I get to my kids' births, I just need to say that nothing can prepare a parent for the experience—including Lamaze classes. When Debra and I attended, they showed us this old footage of a class shot in the mid-sixties. A few hippie couples in bell-bottoms and beads sat around cross-legged giving their warm and fuzzy take on childbirth. They're all waxing mystical, and then the moderator, a crew-cut straight man, asks one flower-power boy, "So tell me, Moonshadow (or whatever his fake Aquarian name was), when your wife, Daffodil, is in transition and in great pain, what are you going to do?" Moonshadow smiles broadly and says, "I'm gonna hold her hand and tell her I love her!" Well, smash cut to Daffodil on a gurney, screaming like she's passing a spiked bowling ball. There's Moonshadow at her side. She looks at hubby and shrieks, "Get the hell away from me!" I whispered to Debra, "If hippie-man takes her hand now, she'll tear off a few of his fingers."

My son Chase was born on April 17, 1987. I remember the night quite well, as my wife and I had eaten a big Mexican dinner, including chili. Debra awoke around 1 A.M. complaining that the food hadn't agreed with her. She figured it was just gas. After four trips to the bathroom, I told her the food was fine, it was probably labor pains. But what do I know? I'm just a stupid male. I suggested she call the doctor, but instead she called her mother. Of course, Mom had no trouble convincing her it wasn't the chili but the child.

At the time, we were living in Manhattan, so we headed for New York Hospital. There must have been a baby boom that night. When we arrived, there were all these guys hanging around the halls by maternity. They were leaning against the walls with their heads down, looking real hangdog. It wasn't the late hour or the lack of sleep—it was because all their wives were having protracted labor and had been screaming at them for thirty-six hours or more. When we walked in, these guys gave me the "welcome to hell" look.

Thankfully, Debra was fully dilated when we got there. Ninety minutes later, without any drugs at all, Chase was born. I walked out of that delivery room looking like I'd won the jackpot. The hangdog heads just dropped lower.

So that was Chase, quick and easy. Amazingly, six years later almost to the day, Debra went into labor with our daughter, Elizabeth. In the middle of the night, Debra's water broke. She wasn't having any contractions at all yet, so we just sort of lounged for a while. After a few hours, she started to feel it, so we got in the car and headed for the hospital in Stamford.

If most births are a marathon, Chase's had been a sprint. I was confident Elizabeth's birth would be a reprise of her older brother's. After getting to the hospital and settling in, with no heavy labor pains yet, the nurse decided to give Debra an IV of Pitocin to get things rolling. I told the nurse that wouldn't be necessary. My suggestion earned me the "I'm a medical professional, don't tell me how to do my job" look from her as she's about to stick the needle into my wife. As soon as she does my wife began SCREAMING with labor pains.

Now the nurse's know-it-all expression fades to terror and she runs away in search of a doctor. Debra continues to scream bloody murder. Meanwhile, I have to keep turning away from Debra to hide my smile and stifle my laughter. Why? I wasn't thinking, "Gee . . . it's great to be male," or taking any pleasure in my wife's pain. For some insane reason I was fixating on the thought that some innocent first-time mommy may well be in the vicinity, hear Debra and pass out with fright—her screams were that bloodcurdling.

Finally, I get my bizarre thoughts in check and a doctor shows up, frantically trying to get his gloves on. Elizabeth begins to appear. Upon somebody's advice, Debra stops screaming and focuses on pushing. Elizabeth pops out.

To this day, Debra calls it her "thirty-seven minutes of hell." And I still have to stifle a laugh.

LOVE CONNECTION

Alicia of Detroit tells how her brother made a love connection, thanks to faith, a baby and a nice sweater.

I was raised Roman Catholic. Heavy on the sin, guilt, G-rated movies and Friday fish. I'm pretty by-the-book in my faith, and plenty of people scoff, but I do believe in divine intervention.

When I found out I was pregnant with my first daughter, my husband was still in the navy, on a submarine. Due to the nature of his mission, he just couldn't get back in time for the birth. At first I was really bummed, but then I realized I was fortunate that he would be back a few days after. Besides, I had a great stand-in, my baby brother, Ed.

Even though we're only two years apart, he's my baby brother and always will be. I feel very protective toward him; and we're as close as siblings can be. A few days before my due date, he stayed over at our house because his place was about an hour away. He wanted to be close by to help.

Those nights were really nice. He'd come home from work, I'd cook something or he'd bring takeout, and we'd catch up and reminisce. About two years before that, he had broken up with some girl, and he was still devastated. I mean inconsolable. Actually, she had dumped him for some scuzzy ex-convict. I always thought, Good riddance to a twenty-two-carat bitch, but Ed didn't see it that way. She was the love of his life and the one that got away. I never understood it. She was probably a sexual athlete. Men are so stupid–even my baby brother.

Well, I had set him up with friends, set him up on blind dates and written personal ads (without telling him). I was determined to fix his broken heart. Nothing worked, and this guy, who had always been the cocky, life-of-the-party chick magnet, was turning into a sad sack.

I lit candles. I even said a novena. Let me tell you he's not just a nice guy, he's great looking. But he was putting out such a negative, loser vibe that nothing worked.

I remember the night I went into labor. We had just finished dinner and were sitting in front of the television shoveling Häagen-Dazs. Suddenly, I felt this pain in my back. "What's wrong?" Ed asked. I told him. "Okay, let's go," he said. I said we didn't have to leave immediately. We should wait until the contractions came closer together. So we just sat around for a couple of hours. Then I really started to cook, so I suggested we head for the hospital, which was a few miles away.

As we're walking to the door, I look at Ed, and he's wearing this old sweatshirt. I said, "Are you going like that?"

"Hey, it's eleven o'clock at night and we're going to a hospital. You want me to rent a tux?"

"Go put on the sweater I bought you for Christmas. You never know who'll you meet." I love bossing him around!

He ran upstairs and came back down in the sweater. Then I told him to take a shave–he had a shadow. So he ran back upstairs to the bathroom, and I felt a really strong contraction.

"Hurry up."

"You want me shaved or you want to have a baby?"

Anyway, he came back down and we got in the car. It was an easy drive to the hospital. We go inside and get comfortable. Then Denise, the labor nurse, comes in, and I swear to God, I saw Ed's heart pounding through his sweater. What a hottie! Suddenly he's Johnny Charm-bomb, and this nurse is reciprocating. Right off, she finds out he's not my husband but my brother. Then that he's single. Once she knows she has a clear shot, she moves in for the kill. "Ed this, Ed that. What do you do? How nice. Where'd you go to school? Do you work out? Do you know so-and-so? Yada yada yada."

She was pushy but in a cute sort of way, and it was so good to see my brother responding–no, make that panting–to a woman again. So I just tried to shut up and let things happen. The weird part is, here I am with my legs up in the air with my privates exposed in the middle of a date! And it was going really, really well. I was actually impressed by some of the comeback lines baby brother had. Still, he was no match for her. She was a nurse but should have been a surgeon–she really knew how to operate!

Once the heavy pushing came, Ed did his duty and focused his attention on me–of course I made him stay by my head–but still you could sense the sparks flying between him and Denise.

Soon I had a 6-pound, 4-ounce baby boy–Paul. Two days later, my husband arrived and we were complete. And Ed and Denise will be married in September.

I'm pretty proud of myself. Novenas, candles, a sexy sweater. Although every time Denise comes over, I feel a little weird, considering how much of me she's seen. I guess it's that Catholic thing.

8

Battle of the TV Moms

Who is the ultimate TV mom, Shirley Partridge
or Carol Brady?
We thought of checking with A. C. Nielsen
to see who pulled the bigger audiences.

Then we considered one of those side-by-side
box charts, listing number of TV offspring,
prestige factor of Mr. Brady (architect) vs.
Shirley Partridge (songbird/single mom),
square footage of TV homes, designer of
TV wardrobe—but that became too ponderous.

So how about this?
A steel-cage nurturing match—first one to
Band-Aid a scraped knee, whip up dinner and
resolve a puppy-love crisis wins the title.

Ready, ladies?

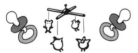

MRS. PARTRIDGE IS PREGNANT!

Shirley Jones of *The Partridge Family* had a five-year reign as America's leading matriarch. She is a performer with remarkable versatility. From *Oklahoma!* to *The Music Man*, and *Drew Carey* to *Melrose Place*, to a thousand club dates in between, Shirley is a rara avis in the entertainment world. She does it all and does it well.

Perhaps she played a mom so convincingly because she is one—three times over. She has some wonderful stories about each birth.

Shaun was first. I was actually pregnant with him for ten months. Jack Cassidy (his father) and I were working then, doing a nightclub act, and we had a packed schedule of bookings way ahead, which went six, eight weeks after the baby was due to arrive. I had gotten so big, and was so overdue, that they decided to induce labor. Well, once they did I was in labor for twelve hours—and it just wasn't happening.

The doctor told us, "His head is so big, and he just doesn't want to come out." He said it looked like a C-section was the only option, which I wasn't happy about because I really wanted to have the experience. So I told him that I wanted to see the birth. I didn't want to be asleep or anything, so they gave me what was called a saddle-block—you were numbed just from the waist down.

They positioned a mirror and I watched everything—I saw that big head come out, then somebody said, "It's a boy!" and I asked if he had his father's dimples. He did, and he also weighed in at a near-colossal 9 pounds, 8 ounces, with lots of long hair. He looked like a two-month-old. The hospital, which was St. John's in Santa Monica, chose to film Shaun in a little movie they made teaching new mothers how to bathe their babies. So he had his first acting job by the time he was a few minutes old!

After Shaun was born, Jack and I had all those club dates to keep, so we took Shaun on the road with us—and I was breast-feeding. Here I am in skimpy little, low-cut dance costumes!

One night, we were in Las Vegas on stage in mid-show, and suddenly, the milk just started to flow and drip right across the stage. I ran behind the curtain and grabbed a towel and decided it was time to switch Shaun to a bottle.

I'll skip ahead to my third son and get back to the second later. They had chosen a date on which to perform the C-section, but two weeks prior I went into labor. And they don't like you to be in labor before a C-section—it makes it more difficult because the baby can get into the birth canal. So I was rushed to the hospital, and what a surprise—Ryan topped Shaun, coming in two weeks ahead of term at a whopping 10 pounds, 8 ounces.

All my boys were by my husband, Jack, who'd had a son—David—before we met. And of course, each time, Jack had hoped for a girl. I was okay with either, although I was becoming pretty adept at raising boys and knowing how to handle them. But it wasn't in the cards—Jack never got his little girl.

Now back to Patrick, my second boy. Audiences may be surprised to learn that I was pregnant throughout most of the filming of *The Music Man*. Three months into the shoot, I found out I was carrying Patrick. I had to tell the director, who almost passed out. They all said, "What are we going to do about this?" So they built a corset, and they kept pulling me in and pulling me in and adding to the petticoats and fringes and bows and raising the waist. Fortunately, it was a period picture and the costumes allowed it. The secret remained safe until one day we were shooting a scene where Robert Preston and I kiss. As he squeezed me, the baby suddenly kicked. Preston's eyes bulged and he said, "What was that?" I had to tell him what it was, so finally the secret was out.

Years later when Patrick was grown, he met Robert Preston. He introduced himself, stuck out his hand and said, "I'm Patrick Cassidy." Preston said, "We've already met!"

HERE'S A STORY OF A LOVELY LADY . . .

Florence Henderson is tied with Shirley Jones for the title
of most famous TV mother, thanks to her half-decade as
mater of *The Brady Bunch*. From her roles as a regular on
The Tonight Show to Carol Brady to feature films, Florence
Henderson has a stellar career. But to kids Barbara, Joseph,
Robert and Elizabeth, she's just . . . "Mom."

I have four children. I was knocked out for the birth of
my first child and don't remember most of it. With the second
one, I was pretty dopey and drifted in and out of consciousness.
So I decided that was enough of that. I wanted to be more in control. I had my third and fourth children naturally.

I always get upset when people say, "Oh boy, I was in so much
pain. What an awful experience." I think it's much easier without
the drugs because you stay in control. With the drugs, you lose
control because you're so tense and afraid. These things add to the
pain.

I taught myself Lamaze and practiced all these different breathing techniques. I really believe that breathing is key to everything—exercise, staying calm and focused. When you lose control,
the pain is endless. I prayed a lot, too.

With each child, I had cravings for salty foods. I'd eat tuna fish
and pickles for breakfast. In those days they didn't make a big deal
about drinking, and I remember every so often I'd crave a sip of
beer and a brownie. Now that's pretty sick, isn't it? I'm not a big
sweets eater and I'm not that crazy about beer, so I don't know
where that came from.

Each labor got a little shorter. During the first one, I had false
labor for three days. That was painful. I had all my children in
New York City, where I was living at the time. Toward the end of
my ninth month with each one, I would get on the Fifth Avenue

bus to try to induce labor. There were so many potholes on the street, I thought maybe they'd jump-start contractions. Once the beginning stages of labor kicked in, I got my hair and nails done. After a few children, you kind of get to know how much you can do before serious labor hits. I had a little time to spare and I didn't want to get to the hospital too early.

I guess for the fourth I waited a little too long. It was really early in the morning and I could feel contractions in my lower back. That means the baby's pretty close to being born. I called my doctor, who said, "Get to the hospital as fast as you can."

I arrived at 6 A.M. There was one nurse available and she was being very formal and calm. My last name was Bernstein at the time, and she would say, "Yes, Mrs. Bernstein. It's okay. The doctor will be here shortly."

Then the doctor came in and he said, "Just a few more contractions and this baby will be here." Well, I had two intense contractions and I said, "The baby's coming. The baby's coming!"

The nurse wheeled me into a delivery room. She was the only person in the room and she was trying to help me crawl onto the table. So calm and so formal before, in the delivery room she was like, "Don't push, Florence. Don't push. Okay, Florence."

The doctor was washing up and he was saying the same things. I panted like a puppy and was doing everything in my power not to push. Finally he came over and said, "Okay. Let's have it." I pushed really hard and there was a head and a shoulder and he goes, "Okay, last chance. What's it going to be?" I said, "It's a little girl." Well, the baby plops out and he goes, "You're right." There was little Lizzie. I had sensed it was a girl all along. I always knew what all my children were going to be. It's just an instinct a mom has.

I'm the youngest of ten children. When I was five, my oldest sister had her first child. So I was around children most of my life. Even as a little girl, I was the mothering type. Although my siblings were all older, I kind of mothered them. So it's funny that I became known as this TV mom because I always considered myself a mom.

It's a totally different ball game when it's your own. What an awesome responsibility! I was a responsible person before the babies were born, but I think motherhood made me much more humble. It lets you know what's really important. What you do in life is a job. A career is just a career. Motherhood is the greatest work of all.

When I got home from the hospital, I didn't get much sleep. And let me tell you, I still don't sleep. Your kids are yours forever and you never let go of them. Even though they're adults now, they're still my babies. I'll always worry about them.

9

Short Takes

A sampling from some doctors, nurses, doulas and parents.

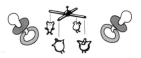

JAMES GANDOLFINI, star of *The Sopranos,* is the father of Michael. He suggests:

*J*ust remember it really changes everything. Life as you know it will never be the same. Unfortunately, you are suddenly forced to become an adult. I wasn't an adult before I had a child. Actually, I wasn't even a child. I was embryonic. Slowly but surely, I'm maturing, thanks to my kid.

RAY ROMANO, star of *Everybody Loves Raymond,* is the father of Alexandra, Joseph and twins Matthew and Gregory. He offers this advice:

*T*his could sound like I'm joking, but I'm actually serious. My advice is to get all the sleep and have all the sex you can before you have your babies. You're gonna find a drastic difference when you have children. Also, during labor, do everything your wife says. Men are all pretty stupid, so you basically just take orders and don't ask questions.

When we had twins, my wife, Anna, and I had to wake up in shifts. We became war buddies. We had to form alliances with each other in order to survive.

NIKKI SIXX of Mötley Crüe looked at his new daughter, Frankie, moments after she was born on January 3, 2001. Here's what he said:

$\mathcal{I}$ told Frankie there's only one thing she can't do in her life . . . date a *rock star.* She agreed.

So I pre-ordered her a pink 2017 BMW for her sixteenth birthday.

She sighed and said, "My daddy's the best."

MELINA KANAKAREDES, star of the television series *Providence* and mom to Zoe, has these words of wisdom for expectant parents:

$\mathcal{I}$ know people say this all the time, but you have to enjoy every second with your children because they do change in a moment's time. It's important for you to become the kid that you know you are, because that's what babies need. You have to be silly, sing songs, all of that.

Before I had my baby, I took Pilates, which is great exercise. If you take a Pilates class early on in your pregnancy, you can do it all the way up to your delivery. I exercised two days before giving birth and I started back at it three weeks later. I feel like I had a really short labor because of exercising. Plus there was no tearing or anything. I was in labor for ten hours—not bad for a first-time mom. I pushed for an hour. Zoe, which means *life* in Greek, came out weighing 7 pounds, 12 ounces. She puts everything in perspective for me.

ED MCMAHON, thirty-year co-host of *The Tonight Show,* helped tuck America in at night. The big Irishman had this remembrance of the birth of his first child:

$\mathcal{M}$y first child, Claudia, was born in a very small hospital in the middle of Florida, my wife's hometown area. I got special leave from the Marine Corps to be around for the arrival. The doctor thought it would be interesting for me to be in the delivery room for the birth. Since I was a fighter pilot, he thought I could handle it. He was extremely mistaken. Seconds before I was about to faint, they moved me into another room, and luckily that room had a bathroom.

I could land on a carrier, but I could not handle the delivery room!

WHAT'S THE MATTER? YOU ALWAYS ENJOY YOUR PROSTATE EXAMS . . .

There was this husband who freaked when he learned what exactly went into an internal exam. As the doctor put on his gloves, the husband turned to me—the nurse—and said, "Why is he doing that?"

I explained that the doctor needed to put his hand inside his wife and feel for the baby.

"I don't want him doing that to my wife. I'll do it!"

At first I thought he was joking and I laughed right at him. But he looked at me and frowned. Then I cleared my throat and said, "I don't think you know what you're really looking for. The doctor's very good at this . . . look, he's already done."

MAYBE SHE HAD THEM BRONZED?

For some reason, this woman just had to deliver her baby standing up. She was wearing really beat-up tennis shoes, which looked a lot worse after her delivery. Afterward, I offered to clean the blood off them. She said, "Leave them alone. Let them dry that way. I want to save them." Sometimes you just don't ask questions, but I still wonder what she had planned for those sneakers.

WE SUPPOSE THAT'S NOT YOUR BABY, EITHER!

One particular patient was really, really loud. She was screaming at the top of her lungs the entire time she was in labor, which was fifteen hours. It was crazy. I couldn't stand it. It was draining me. It took everything in my power not to walk out on her. She gave me a migraine with her whining and screaming. At one point, her husband just left, claiming he was getting some fresh air, but he came back two hours later. By then, he didn't care if he missed the birth.

He'd try to calm her, but that would make her scream even more. She'd say things like, "How can you ask me to calm down when you have no idea what this is like? You have no idea what pain is. You did this to me!"

Then after she gave birth, she says to me, "My God, that woman down the hall was screaming bloody murder." She really had no idea.

I could barely move. My ears were ringing. I didn't even tell her. I just looked at her husband, who was more exhausted than she was. She turned to him and goes, "Let's order a pizza."

SAY, ISN'T THAT A GLADIATOR NAME?

I was a labor nurse for this mom, and her water had just broken. The doc mentioned something about "meconium" (the baby's first bowel movement) being in the fluid, but this woman had no idea what it was. She and I were talking a little bit later, and she said she had heard a cool name for her son while waiting for his arrival. She wanted to name him *Meconium!!!*

Another nurse and I set her straight, but we had a really hard time keeping a serious face while explaining this to her!

PIANO STOOL OR MILKING STOOL?

This woman had been in labor for a really, really long time. Finally, she was nearing the end. But she was giving these little, feeble pushes. We kept telling her to push harder. So she put a little more uumph into it.

The midwife was standing right at her legs and suddenly got very joyful. "I see the head! I see the head! The head's coming!" We all got excited and sprang into action. There was this flurry of motion. Then the midwife sighed and said in her very proper British accent, "Oh no . . . it's just a stool."

We just started laughing and laughing. We were killing ourselves with laughter. The woman delivering the baby neither heard nor noticed. She was in her own world. Her husband chuckled. I wonder if he ever told her.

SAY IT LIKE YOU MEAN IT!

A woman in labor kept screaming and crying, pleading, "I can't do this. I need drugs! Drugs! DRUGS!!!!!!!!"

Throughout her pregnancy, she had been very adamant about the whole natural childbirth thing, but there she was, screaming for drugs. I looked at her husband, who all along had been very skeptical about her ability to endure pain. So I thought he'd just nod and say, "Sure. Give her the drugs." Instead, he studied his wife. I went over to him. "You know your wife better than anyone. What's your take on this?"

He stared at his wife for a long time. Then he turned to me and said, "She's not asking hard enough."

I couldn't believe it! She seemed pretty sincere to me. I said, "Okay. If that's your take on it." A little while later she gave birth and was very relieved to have had a drug-free delivery. "See? I knew I could handle it," she said.

NEXT TIME SHE'LL HAVE A ROLL OF DIMES
IN HER FIST

My wife is a very mild-mannered person, but during the birth of our son, she became very angry and mean. We had gone through Lamaze classes, so I remembered the instructor had talked about this. She was yelling at me for every little thing. Finally, I bent over, stroked her hair and very lovingly said, "It's okay. We learned about this in Lamaze. You're transitioning."

I thought I was being the understanding, sensitive male. The next thing I knew, she belted me right in the face. "They didn't teach that in Lamaze, did they," she said.

MEMO TO MR. EXCITEMENT

Toward the end of her labor, this patient was getting out of control. She was screaming and cursing at her husband. "It's all your fault! It's all your fault," this woman said over and over. Finally the nurse had enough of it. "You know, honey, it takes two to get to this spot here." Well, the woman just glared at the nurse and screamed, "I WAS ASLEEP THE WHOLE TIME!"

I MEANT THAT IN THE GOOD SENSE

This woman came into the emergency room complaining of severe stomach pains. She thought she had food poisoning or a virus. "You're not sick," the doctor says. "You're in labor."

Well, the woman and her husband were in shock. They had no idea she was even pregnant. The doctor said, "Couldn't you tell?" The husband looked at him and said, "I just thought she was starting to look like her mother."

WANNA KNOW WHAT COMES BETWEEN ME AND MY CALVINS?

A woman came into the emergency room screaming that she was having a baby. When most women do this, they're still hours and hours away from actually giving birth. But this woman was screaming her lungs out, and then she stopped and a wave of relief passed over her and she smiled. She had delivered the baby! It was caught in the legs of her underpants. Mother and baby were fine. And her underwear didn't even have a rip. We joked that this baby should be an underwear model.

OKAY, WE'LL KEEP A LINE OPEN TO THE GOVERNOR

*W*e hook up the fetal monitor to this woman pregnant with her first child. The monitor goes inside the woman and attaches to the baby's head.

Anyway, the woman's bags of water are dripping. She becomes convinced that she's going to get electrocuted. She tells me I'm inept and I don't know what I'm doing. She's screaming and screaming, "I'm being electrocuted. I'm dying. I can feel the shock running through my body. Help!" The baby's head is practically out of her, but she doesn't notice. She's too busy imagining she's near death.

HERE'S SOMETHING FOR YOUR
ATTENTION DEFICIT, DOC

*T*his woman had a two-year-old who had been born by C-section. So this time around, she was very committed to having a drug-free, vaginal birth.

She was pushing in the typically American position of semi-sitting, which usually puts the doctor at an advantage but can give the woman bad leg cramps. And she got some pretty intense ones. The first time she just said, "Oh, it's cramping, it's cramping." I was able to massage it out.

The doctor was standing, all scrubbed up, between her legs, not really paying any attention to her, when suddenly she said, "A CRAMP!" Her leg shot out in front of her and knocked the doctor in the chin. He flew backward and landed on his butt. Needless to say, he paid attention to her leg cramping after that.

PUSH, BUT NOT QUITE THAT HARD

This mother was pushing really, really hard. Suddenly, there was this loud pop like a bottle of champagne opening. I've been a nurse for a long time, but I've never heard anything like it before. The next thing, water was just exploding out of her like a geyser and the doctor was drenched in it. It gushed out and practically drowned him—his head and gown were covered. The water hit the wall, too.

We all laughed. The doctor laughed the hardest. Someone handed him a towel and he wiped his face. I don't think people realize how much water's in there.

OKAY, BUT I'LL BE THINKING ABOUT LIPSTICK LESBIANS

My sister's water broke at 5 P.M. on Saturday. By 3 P.M. on Sunday, she was still only three centimeters dilated. My sister was using a midwife and the birth was taking place at an old schoolhouse. Well, her husband was this very shy man and the whole concept of midwives was new to him. He was very nervous.

When the midwife checked my sister and saw that she was only at three centimeters, she took Tom around the corner. My other sister and I were in a nearby room so we heard the midwife say, "Well. Ahh. We need some help from you. We're going to need your semen." You could just hear the silence and imagine poor Tom's face draining of any color.

My sister and I just covered our mouths—we were laughing so

hard. Then we ran out of the house and into town. We went to an ice cream shop and drank milk shakes as slowly as possible. "You think they're done yet?" we asked each other. Finally, when we imagined they had to be finished, we left.

We came back and the poor guy's sitting on the steps with his head in his hands. He was so embarrassed. There were his two sisters-in-law and his mother-in-law, and all of us were looking at him like, "We know what you guys were doing."

But prostaglandins in the semen really soften the cervix and get labor going. Within a few hours my sister was six centimeters. Then she quickly went to ten and pushed the baby out in forty-five minutes. I think Tom was pretty proud of himself. But after that he could never look at us without blushing.

PUT A BOWLING BALL IN THERE—I WANNA FEEL LIKE I DID SOMETHING!

This woman was stuck at eight centimeters, so the doctor suggested she take a shower. When she came out, she just stood in the middle of the room. She looked at her mom and said, "Mommy, I'm having a contraction." And her mother went over to her and gave her this big bear hug and goes, "There, there."

From that moment on, every time she had a contraction, she wanted a hug. Just as a contraction would begin, she'd go, "Hug me." So we all took turns. There was the mother, husband, nurse and me, her doula. We sat in a circle. Every four minutes, one of us would move toward her and put our arms around her from behind. We'd just hold her through the whole contraction. We hugged her for two hours.

Then the nurse said, "The baby's there. You have to push the baby out." Of course, like all women, the first time she didn't do it right. She didn't do it right the second or third time, either. By the fourth push, the baby's head was out. By the fifth push, the baby was completely out. The nurse put the baby on the mother, but she didn't seem to notice. She was still pushing. The nurse goes, "That's your baby on your stomach." And she goes, "I'm not finished." She couldn't believe it wasn't more painful.

HOW MUCH GODIVA WAS THAT?

There was a blond, blue-eyed mother and a blond, blue-eyed father. I kept telling them, "Oh, your baby's going to be beautiful. You're going to have this little blond, blue-eyed baby." Me and my big mouth.

The baby was beautiful—and black. The father just looked at me with his mouth hanging open. "Is that baby black, or is it after-birth?"

I said, "You'll have to ask your wife that."

They worked it out. They even had another baby—with blond hair and blue eyes.

I heard the mother didn't know what to tell her own mom. So she told her she ate a lot of chocolate during the pregnancy.

The mother believed it. People believe what they want to believe.

ISN'T THIS THE START OF A LETTER TO *PENTHOUSE?*

I had just become a labor nurse. There was this one patient who had been in the hospital in labor for twenty-four hours. She was in a lot of pain, but she hadn't dilated enough to push. I knew it would be a few more hours. She didn't want any medication, but I wanted her to take a nap. I sent her husband out to get something to eat. I was in the room with her and pushing on her back to alleviate some of the pain.

Anyway, to do it better, I actually get behind her in the bed and apply pressure. Well, I had been doing a double shift and was exhausted. The next thing, I wake up and her husband's staring down at me. I'm mortified! I jump out of the bed. "Don't go. My wife's in bed with a woman. That's always been my fantasy," he says.

I'M READY FOR MY CLOSE-UP

This woman was about to have the baby in the house. I called the paramedics. She was pushing and she had her shorts on, so I told her to take her shorts off.

Then I told her the paramedics were on the way and suddenly she headed for the bathroom and started putting on makeup. I said, "What are you doing?" She said, "I can't let them see me this way." She was putting on mascara and crouching in pain. She was pushing while applying lipstick. I told her, "They don't care." She goes, "I CARE. I won't go out in public looking like this!" She stayed in the bathroom until she had her makeup exactly the way she wanted it.

?YBAB EHT SAW GIB WOH

One morning in my eighth month, I woke up with this excruciating pain. I called my obstetrician, who said that the soft tissue between my left and right pelvis was inflamed. He told me there was really nothing I could do.

The pain became so severe that I found it impossible to walk. The angle of the bone goes backward so that putting my feet forward resulted in agony. However, when I walked backward, it wasn't painful at all. So for the last month of my pregnancy, I'd do everything backward. I'd go to the supermarket with my daughter and she'd direct me. "Okay, Mom, make a left there. Take two more steps and you'll be right at the bread." I actually became quite adept at backward walking, although I got a lot of peculiar looks. Strangely enough, no one ever said anything. If they had, I would have told them I was pledging a sorority, and really made them wonder.

When labor started, I walked backward to my car. Christopher was born five hours later. When I visited him in the hospital nursery I was able to walk forward. Although by then it felt a little odd.

I SAID LIGHT TOAST!

*W*hen you've had as many C-sections as I have, you know the drill. I was in for my sixth scheduled cesarean. I'm on the table and the doctor's doing his thing. As I'm lying there, the horrible stench of burning flesh wafts through the air, so I know the doctor has cut me open.

I go, "Now there's a lovely smell." The doctor looks a little perplexed and asks for an explanation. I say, "I can smell my burning flesh. It's disgusting."

The doctor laughs. "I haven't opened you yet. That's not burning flesh. That's the cafeteria downstairs. It's breakfast."

I say, "Remind me to avoid the cafeteria."

10

The Do-It-Yourselfers

There's nothing like Yankee ingenuity. These moms and dads raise self-reliance to an art form.

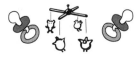

OKAY, YOU HELPED DELIVER A BABY . . . BUT DID YOU SELL ANY TERM LIFE TO THE PARAMEDICS?

Zoltan Gombas, an insurance executive from Oakland, New Jersey, shows how fate laughs at those who think they're prepared.

It was dinnertime and my wife, Gina, was about to bite down on some eggs when the fork falls to the floor. She looks at me and says, "My water just broke."

We had everything planned for this moment. I say, "Cool. I'll call Francine." Francine, her sister, was slated to baby-sit our son, Andrew, who was not yet two. Gina goes, "Tell her not to rush. We have time."

We were very calm. Partly because Andrew had been induced two weeks after his due date. Then he took another six hours to arrive, even though they gave Gina some Pitocin to quicken the pace. We assumed we had loads of time.

Gina goes upstairs to take a shower and pack her bags. I play with Andrew for a while, then I check on Gina. She's grimacing in pain, gripping the sink and blow-drying her hair all at once. I ask, "Gina, why do you look like that?" She gives a quick smile. "I'm okay. I'm fine," she says, but she's gritting her teeth.

Francine arrives, so I go outside to warm up the car. I turn it around and back it up in the driveway for an easy exit. I leave the motor running and go into the house for my wife. The minute I walk in the door, Francine hands me the phone. Gina's next to her bent over in pain. I grab the phone. "Who's this?" I say. "I really don't have time to take a phone call."

"It's 911" was the answer.

"Gina, 911!!!!!!!!!! Get in the car. Let's go."

Gina looks at me. Let me explain my wife to you: She's a very quiet person. We've been together for eight years and she never raises her voice to me. The first time I heard her yell at the dog, I was shocked. Anyway, she looks at me and screams:

"I'M NOT GOING TO MAKE IT TO THE CAR!"

My wife never exaggerates. She's no drama queen; she's as stoic as they come. When she says she's not going to make it, I know she isn't going to make it. I start speaking into the phone.

Ron, the cop on the line, tells me the first thing I have to do is get my wife on the floor. "If that baby comes out, it's going to fall headfirst."

I tell Gina to get on the floor, but she's gripping the banister. She looks at me. "I can't move," she says.

"Gina, please get on the floor."

"I can't."

Ron hears this. "You've got to get her on the floor right now!"

Gina won't budge, so I run up to her and tackle her to the floor. I bear all the weight, so I fall backward on the hardwood floor with the phone still stuck in the crook of my neck. I was pretty proud that I still had that phone. I bang my head pretty hard.

All this is too much for Sandy, our seventy-five-pound golden retriever. She thinks it's playtime. And she jumps on top of us and licks our faces. Andrew, who's at the top of the stairs, thinks he's missing out on the fun. He's shaking the iron gate he's behind, screaming, "Mommy Mommy Mommy. Downstairs now! Mommy Mommy Mommy. Downstairs now!" Francine's with him, but she's in a state of shock. She's crying with a vacant look in her eyes.

"Play with your aunt," Gina barks through her teeth.

I jump up, grab Sandy with one hand and shove her into a bedroom. My sister-in-law is throwing every towel we have in the house down to me. I grab a few and head toward Gina. That's when I see the baby's head. It's already starting to come out.

I have a conversation with myself. I say, "This is a defining moment of your life. No matter what, this is going to happen. You can't stop it." I sell insurance, and in my job I get uptight sometimes. I say to myself that I will never again worry about something stupid for as long as I live. I say this again and again. "I will never worry about stupid things for as long as I live."

I remember the doctor had pressed on Gina's stomach a little bit the first time around. I tell Gina to push and I press down a bit. All of a sudden, the baby just pops out. I catch it and hold it in my arms. I'm sitting there in a daze with this baby. I can't move.

The cop on the line is talking. At first I don't hear him. The sound is muffled and distant. "What's going on? What's going on? Hello?"

"The baby's out."

"Congratulations! What is it, Daddy?"

I couldn't believe it. I'm worrying that my wife and kid might have died and he's asking the sex of my child. I had no idea. I couldn't move.

"What is it, Daddy?"

I look. A girl. I tell Ron. I'm still in a daze. But I wrap her in a towel and put her on my wife's chest. Suddenly the cops come in. They throw me out of the way, dive down on the floor with my wife and start checking the baby. Two minutes later, two ambulances pull up and my house is crowded with strangers.

One of the emergency medical technicians tells me I should take a picture. I tell him I have no idea where a camera is. "There's one around your neck," he informs me. I didn't even realize it. When I had put my things together, I had hung a camera around my neck and completely forgotten about it. I clicked some photos. Then I cut the cord. My hands were still shaking.

I drove alone to the hospital, following the ambulance carrying my wife and new baby, Stephanie. The car was nice and warm. After I visited both of them, I headed home and cleaned the floors. It was about two thirty in the morning. Even though it was thirty degrees out, I went out on the deck with a huge glass of vodka and a cigar. I finished both and then headed to bed. It was then that I realized I had a huge bump on my head from tackling my wife to the floor. It was starting to sting.

GIRLS JUST WANNA HAVE BABIES

Cyndi Lauper exploded onto the music scene in the eighties with a string of chart-topping hits like "True Colors," "Girls Just Wanna Have Fun," "She-Bop" and "Time After Time." After playing the biggest of venues to SRO crowds, Cyndi claims her best performance was when she introduced her son—with husband, actor David Thornton—to the world.

I was set on having natural childbirth. And once I make up my mind that I'm going to do something, you might as well understand that's how it will be—come hell or high water, I will do it.

I was three days late and I was a little nervous because after a certain point, the doctor wants to induce you if you're late. I didn't want any drugs in my system. My girlfriend told me if I tweaked my nipples, I could induce myself. So I'm sitting on a bench at home, massaging my nipples and watching the most ridiculous movie on television, *Bella Mafia*. I just watched and tweaked. Watched and tweaked.

I sat there wondering if I should go out dancing that night with some friends, but a sharp pain in my lower stomach answered the question for me. I wasn't going anywhere. I was finally in labor. It was about 9 P.M. on November 18, 1997.

I got kind of weird. I didn't really want David, my husband, to see me in pain. So I sequestered myself in the bathroom. I'd go from the shower to the bathtub to the toilet. I was throwing up a lot. I filled the tub with warm water to help with the pain. I didn't want to get to the hospital too early because they practically line you up in the parking lot for your epidural.

The birthing teacher said that when you first go into labor try to get some sleep. But that's just one of the silliest things I've ever heard. How can you sleep? You're in labor! Duh!

I practically sat in the tub all night. I played a lot of music. One of my birthing songs was "Disco Inferno," which I wound up recording. I listened to a lot of ABBA as well as the song by Sylvester, "You Make Me Feel Mighty Real." They were kind of powerful songs that helped me deal with the pain. I also sang a song for my baby, which I recorded in 1994, called, "Come on Home." It was a sweet moment. Every now and then, David would venture into the bathroom with toast, which I'd devour and immediately throw up. Then he'd make some more. He'd tell me so-and-so was on the phone. I'd just say, "I can't talk. I can't talk. Are you crazy? I can't talk."

I didn't want to get out of the tub. The doctor begged me to come to the hospital. David couldn't find us a car service in Manhattan, but finally he got a Town Car from a place called Diva Limousines. We thought that was pretty funny.

I admit that when I got to the hospital, I was screaming in pain. I had already been in labor for nearly fourteen hours. We had practically packed up the apartment in my bags. So while I was in the delivery room, poor David was bringing up my bags. When we got to the hospital it was 11:25 A.M. and I was fully dilated. A nurse said to David, "Pal, leave this stuff. Your wife is delivering your baby. You're going to miss it." He raced to the room. I don't know if he was procrastinating. I wanted David in the room with me, but there were times he couldn't look. He didn't want to cut the cord, but he was the first to hold the baby. They have an incredible bond.

Declyn Wallace Lauper Thornton was born at 12:35 P.M. on November 19, 1997, weighing 8 pounds, 15 ounces. The kid came out with his hands up like "Power to the people." When I was first pregnant, I was convinced the baby would be a girl. Then one night, a few months into the pregnancy, I had a dream it was a boy. Then I just knew.

Up until I was seven months pregnant, I was on tour opening for Tina Turner. I'm glad I worked because I would have had too much time to think and get nervous. But it wasn't easy. I'd have a bucket on each side of the stage in case I got sick. I always get nervous when I'm about to perform, but the pregnancy just exacerbated the nauseous feeling. Once I was onstage singing, though, I was fine. Singing always calms me and it's so good for the baby.

There were some really magical moments on tour, where I'd say, "Declyn, that's Tina Turner singing." Before I'd go onstage, I'd say, "Okay, kid, hold on to Mommy. Here we go. This is our first song." I never felt alone with this little guy inside me.

We always said if he had my temperament and his father's singing voice, Declyn would be in trouble. But he has the sweetest little voice. He loves music. He has a little drum kit. He likes baseball, basketball and hockey. Sometimes we have to call him Larry Bird or Mark Messier. It depends on what he's into that day. He has all these little starting lineup action figures. These are today's little toy soldiers, I guess.

He's an amazing little guy. In the hospital, I wouldn't let him out of my sight at all. The nurses wanted to put him in the nursery, but I wouldn't let them. When we got home, he slept between David and me. People said, "Aren't you worried you might crush him?"

But I just don't understand sticking a baby in another room with a monitor. You're listening to him all night anyway. For the first few months, I was up every two hours nursing him. There was no such thing as sleep.

The funny thing is that I thought having the baby was the whole thing, but after that is when it all starts. I've decided that the terrible twos are nothing. Three is a lot more terrible. But Declyn's actually a great little guy.

FAUX XENA

Teresa Howard from Lawrenceville, Georgia, is a professional doula—a woman who offers support to laboring moms. She tells this tale of her encounter with a mother with an interesting self-image.

$\mathcal{P}$aula had already given birth—with the aid of epidurals and other assorted drugs—to three children. She wanted the fourth one to be natural. She was very adamant about it. I don't think she had any idea what giving birth felt like. She was a quiet woman. A Mormon. The more babies, the better, is their philosophy. Well, I have to be honest with you; I didn't know if she had it in her. A lot of women who've been drugged up say they want a natural birth. When they feel those strong contractions, though, that's another story.

As a doula, I show up at the house when labor begins and stay with my clients through delivery. Paula calls me at 3:30 A.M. At 6:15 A.M., we leave the house for the hospital. Just as we're out the door, she vomits on the steps of the front porch. I realize that we're cutting it close. I put a towel under her seat in the car just to be safe. We make it to the hospital in about twenty-five minutes. By now, her contractions are two minutes apart.

We finally get to the room and the nurse starts preparing an IV. Well, I knew this mom wanted it all natural and she wouldn't stand for any IV. I tell the dad to say something to the nurse, but he's sitting in a chair reading *Newsweek*. Anyway, I'm telling the doctor that Paula will freak out if she even sees the IV, and that's when she screams at the top of her lungs, "NO IV!" The nurse jumps back, terrified. My ears ring.

"If you try again, I swear she'll bite you," I say.

So with that, there was no IV.

By 6:50 A.M., the mom is at ten centimeters. By 7:20 A.M., I tell Paula she can do some light pushing.

"Shut up!"

"This will really help you get used to the feel of things," I suggest.

"Shut up! Just cut the baby out! Get this baby out of me right now!"

I finally convince her to start pushing. She only needs to push a few times and her daughter is born at 7:33 A.M. She weighs 9 pounds, 3 ounces. They name her Sabrina.

The baby's on her chest and Paula's really content. But suddenly her eyes go wide. She looks horrified. "What's this?" she says. I think she believes she's having another baby. I calmly tell her it's the placenta being expelled.

"That is the grossest thing I have ever felt," she says.

She takes a look at it. "That is the grossest thing I have ever seen."

She gets all cleaned up. She's feeding the baby. She's grinning from ear to ear. She's ecstatic. The doctor's about to leave the room, but he stops and looks at Paula. "You did a really good job."

Well, Paula just squints at him. She speaks very slowly and emphatically. "Doctor, I did not do a very good job. I did an awesome job."

Then she raises her arm like she's holding a sword. "I am Xena, the birth warrior."

The doctor's eyes widen. He looks over at me. "Uh-huh."

Anyway, ever since this baby, Paula is a different person. Her friends say she's more confident and outgoing since natural childbirth. She feels she can do anything. I hear she'll occasionally raise her arm and exclaim, "I'm Xena!"

NOW *THIS* IS XENA!

She's punched out more bad guys than John Wayne. Her skills with sword and shield are matchless. Lucy Lawless, star of *Xena*, was quite the warrior princess when it came to the home birth of her son, Julius, in Auckland, New Zealand. Rob Tapert, *Xena*'s executive producer as well as Lucy's husband, gives his take on the experience:

From the start, Lucy was very adamant that she wanted a home birth. I thought it was just a passing fancy, but as we got closer to the due date, I realized she wasn't going to change her mind. She decided to give birth at our house in a tank of water. I was like, "Well, okay." Although this was very normal in Auckland, it all sounded pretty weird to me.

One morning, Lucy woke up at four. She looked at me and declared, "This baby's going to be here by noon." But we had about twenty-five workmen stomping in and out of the house building a pool and a garden. I think that ended up inhibiting Lucy because a full day goes by and nothing much happens. Lucy does have some contractions but not full labor. That night we fall asleep, and few hours later Lucy tells me that the contractions are coming closer. She asks me to time them.

"They're about seven minutes apart," I tell her. I start timing again, but suddenly the minute hand goes fuzzy and I fall back asleep. Lucy wakes me up three hours later.

"Now it's time to get real," she says. It was very *Xena*-esque of her.

I guess I was a bit nervous, but I was so excited. Lucy says I padded around the house looking for things I thought I desperately needed, but now I have no idea what they were. We called the midwife, who got there at four. She put Lucy in this water tank that's about three feet deep and six feet across. Supposedly, the water lessens the weight of the baby pushing against your abdomen. It helps alleviate the labor pains.

At 6 A.M., I wake up eleven-year-old Daisy, who is Lucy's daughter from a previous marriage. She is thrilled to be in the room with her mom.

As the baby's coming down the birth canal, the midwife tells Lucy, "Now you can feel the baby's head." She tells Lucy to put her fingers inside her and feel. Lucy goes, "Oh my God, the head's right there. It's coming!" The midwife turns to me and goes, "Okay, do you want to feel the baby's head?" After I do, Lucy turns to Daisy and says, "Do you want to feel your little brother's head?"

Well that was just too much. Daisy screams, "No!" And she tears out of the room. The thought of putting her hand anywhere near her mother's vagina spun her out of control!

But it was time for the baby to come out. The midwife took a picture about a second before the baby emerged. You could see from Lucy's face that she was in a tremendous amount of pain. Then the midwife took a picture about a minute later. The baby had been born and there was nothing but elation on Lucy's face. It's amazing the sensations that race through you. Agony one moment, joy the next. Incredible. And once the baby had been born, Lucy could barely remember the pain. She says it was no big deal. She's a true warrior.

For a while, Lucy just cuddles with him in the tub. I cut the cord. Then the midwife hands the baby to me and tells me to pull up my T-shirt so he could snuggle against my skin.

Julius Robert Bay Tapert was born on October 16, 1999, at 7:01 P.M. He weighed 8 pounds, 13 ounces. He kind of looks like me. Even in the sonogram at seventeen weeks, we joked that he had my profile.

It was remarkable. I walked the little guy around the house. I showed him the kitchen and the living room. Then I introduced him to the dog, who was completely puzzled. He couldn't figure out what this new creature was doing in his house. He may have been a little jealous. Then Julius and I stood at the window and I explained the lay of the land to him. It was my way of welcoming him home.

SOME ASSEMBLY REQUIRED

Mike Anderson, an artist from Southern California, always thought of himself as a pretty handy guy—until he tried to assemble his daughter's crib.

*M*argaret went into labor at around 3 A.M. At first she thought it was more of the back pains she'd been experiencing for a few weeks. Then, when they intensified, we knew it was show-time. The drive to the hospital was through streets that were utterly deserted. When we arrived around 4 A.M., we were so calm the night nurse thought we were there to have labor induced.

A few hours later, Jennifer arrived. In no time, Margaret was ensconced in a nice room, nursing the baby. I got out of there as soon as I could, because the one thing I'd failed to do before labor began was assemble the crib. It was still sealed in its cardboard shipping carton—the one with the big letters proclaiming EASY ASSEMBLY.

Confidently, I slit the brown packing tape and opened the flaps of the box. Inside, glaring at me—no, mocking me in their twinkling chromed brilliance—were enough nuts, bolts, springs, screws and assorted hardware to reinforce the Eiffel Tower.

This must be easier than it looks, I thought. So I opened the instruction manual. The illustrations were Jackson Pollock thumbnails—captioned in Cyrillic! Christ! Should I call my younger brother? Hell no, that would give him a lifetime edge in our sibling rivalry.

"Screw you," I seethed at the buffet of parts. Over the years I'd assembled bikes, repaired fishing reels, tuned up cars and done brake jobs, masonry and concrete work. "C'mon—a crib is only a four-sided box and foam mattress. Instructions are always written by morons! I'll figure this out."

But it was more than a four-sided box. This was a Baby Brougham Double Dropside Delux with four-position spring brackets and Kaiserhead X-D bolts with Day4Nite-bed conversion rails. Huh?

I checked the clock in the spare bedroom/nursery: 6:45 P.M.– this shouldn't take more than an hour. By midnight, I had two sides attached, but they hinged at about a 110-degree angle, and a good two inches separated the tops from being flush. My eyes were seeing double. Thinking eight hours' sleep might improve my skill level, I sacked out, setting the alarm for 8 A.M. That would give me about three and a half hours to finish the job and leave for the hospital. Margaret and Jennifer were expecting Daddy at noon.

The next morning I wolfed down two bowls of Frosted Flakes. Fueled by enough sucrose to trigger a diabetic coma, I faced that crib with the balls of Tony the Tiger.

The instruction manual was laid out in ten easy steps–last night I'd blown through . . . two? Jeez! Let's see–L-brackets, stabilizer bars, gate shoes, angle brackets, I-bolts, bolt slugs, the hip bone's connected to the thigh bone, the thigh bone's connected to the . . . Shit!

Sweating like a hippo in a steeplechase, I finally had all four sides connected, but they sagged and listed in a weird rhomboid configuration. Crawling underneath with my flashlight and reading glasses, I lay on my back trying to diagnose what was no doubt some design error perpetrated by the *freaking moron who engineered this piece of shit!*

After shouting this indictment loud enough to be heard by neighbors–in the next zip code–I had a eureka moment. It was the L-brackets! I had inverted the L-brackets! But since they were fastened by slotted Phillips wood screws–the kind that go in easily but once removed leave a useless hole that leaks sawdust in perpetuity–I needed to drill fresh holes.

Ten fifty-eight A.M. If I can knock this off in twenty minutes, I can still be on time to pick up Margaret and the baby.

I raced to the garage to get the trusty Black & Decker ³/₈-inch drill. Months before, in preparation for the arrival of our first child, I had spent a weekend sorting a ten-year accumulation of garage crap. Everything had been thrown out, hung from a Peg-Board or fastened to the overhead joists. The only things touching the floor were the tires of the Toyota. Way up on a shelf, behind a hanging shovel and rake, sat the drill. I removed the garden tools, set them aside, got up on tippy-toe and grabbed the drill. While reaching to replace the shovel, I stepped on the rake. The last thing I remember was the big, thick wooden handle of that rake whooshing up to smack my forehead with the same sound Sammy Sosa's Louisville Slugger makes on those white leather spheres.

I woke up in the ambulance. The rake had split my forehead and knocked me cold. When I landed on the garage floor, the back of my noggin hit pretty hard and sustained a concussion. Tom, the guy across the street, found me lying in a pond of my own type AB negative and, when he couldn't rouse me, dialed 911.

The paramedics were fast drivers, and they got me to the hospital at about 12:05. Not too late! My wife, sitting in a wheelchair with Jennifer on her lap, watched with amazement and horror as I, strapped to a gurney, looking like I'd lost a fight with a Rototiller, was wheeled past her.

"Hi, girls! Daddy had a little accident, but the crib is almost ready," I mumbled through blood-caked lips.

Eight stitches and several ice packs later, we three rode home—in a taxi. That night Jennifer slept in a bassinet. It had been purchased fully assembled.

WHEEL OF FORTUNE!

Marion O'Connor, a mom from a suburb of Rochester, New York, had Pat Sajak and Vanna White for labor coaches.

$\mathcal{I}$ was on my third child. The first two had been delivered in the hospital, just like everyone else. But the hospital thing didn't thrill my husband or me. All that stainless steel and tile, the commotion of doctors and nurses, bright lights, loudspeakers making announcements just seems like a pretty jarring way for a baby to enter the world. Especially when you consider how they've spent the first nine months. Of course, that's just our take on it. The babies are probably oblivious. Nonetheless, I wanted to have my third in our quiet, cozy home.

We'd moved way up here from the city years before and never looked back. We're not survivalists, but we enjoy being as independent as possible. In the summer, we grow a lot of our own vegetables. Bill hunts and fishes. Of course, that's not how we make a living, but we do enjoy going it alone. We have our own power generator and so on, and there's very little Bill can't fix. We have a nice, quiet life, very close to nature. We don't have to deal with rush-hour traffic, road rage, crime, noisy neighbors—and we like that just fine.

Someone recommended a midwife who lived a few miles away. She was very competent and sweet and had terrific references that seemed to be well deserved.

Well, right on my due date, a whopper of a winter storm blew in. And way up here, when it goes like that, things can stop pretty fast and stay that way for a while. Around two o'clock, the view from our porch looked like an arctic whiteout. It was fierce. I started feeling back pain and knew the show was about to start. I called the midwife and she said she would be over right away.

About an hour later, I called the midwife and got her answering machine. Bill asked if he should go outside and put the chains on the four-by-four. But you couldn't even see the driveway, and forget about the road. Even if we had wanted to go to the hospital, there's no way we could have. It seemed like fate, or at least the weather, wanted this baby born at home.

I started to feel quite a bit of pain. I walked around, squatted down, stretched and did all sorts of things to try to stifle the pain—things I had rehearsed with the midwife. Bill was great. He walked with me, talked and rubbed my back.

Our two children, Jason and Samantha, were about eight and ten then, and they were wonderful. They watched everything and tried to help. I remember Samantha kept asking if she could make me a sandwich. She was so cute. But all I wanted was for her to make the roads clear so the midwife could get there.

The only place that I felt comfortable was on the couch in the living room. Bill got me all set on the couch with pillows, towels and sheets, then he built a nice fire in the fireplace. It was dark out now. Looking at the windows, all you could see was the snow gathering at the corners of the panes.

My water broke, and that's when the pain became excruciating. I had had no idea. Stainless steel and tiles and painkilling drugs suddenly seemed more attractive than a cozy, quiet home birth. I was in agony. I needed some distraction, and I told the kids to turn on the television. *Wheel of Fortune* was on. The kids loved the show, so Bill said, "Let's all watch it while Mommy has this baby."

I tried to do what the midwife had said and focused on something while I counted and breathed, and that silly spinning wheel was the perfect thing. For a while, it seemed like it was in sync with my contractions. Some contestant would reach over and spin, then I'd stare at it and listen to that spinning sound while I breathed and counted through the contractions. The audience would applaud me for getting through that one. Then the whole thing began again. Between Vanna's letter-turning strolls, I remember looking at her trim little body and thinking, "I used to be built like that," then POW, another contraction, to bring me back to the job at hand.

Of course, all through this, Bill was coaching, holding my

hand. Well, just about the time some guy was trying to solve the final puzzle, little Steven was born. He was beautiful.

The phone rang, and it was the midwife. She was still stuck in the storm. She talked Bill through the umbilical cord, placenta and so on. Bill cleaned the baby up and gave him to me. Someone shut the television off. We all sat together in front of the fire. I started nursing the baby.

Jason said, "Look, the snow stopped!" A brilliant, almost full moon lit the view from the window, while the five of us snuggled together. It was all that we hoped it would be.

WARM BLANKETS

Brian Quinn, an instructor/paramedic at Gold Cross Ambulance in Rochester, Minnesota, has a tale about his first "field delivery."

It was five or six years back, when I was working for another company in another state. It was an overcast winter day, and we got a "hurry up quick" call from a teenage boy a few miles away. His sister was going into labor, and he was going into an altered state.

My partner had already been a paramedic for a number of years, but I was pretty green so I readily agreed to let him do the heavy lifting while I assisted.

We arrived at the home very quickly, charged up the walkway and rang the bell. The door flew open and here was this kid—I later found out he was seventeen, but he looked much younger. He was so excited. He reminded me of the old Daffy Duck cartoons, when Daffy would become so flummoxed, his head would spin around while he flapped his wings to a blur. This young fellow was really wound up that tight.

Turns out his sister was house-sitting their parents' home. Her husband was on a business trip several states away, and the brother was her only family nearby. He quickly took us to the bathroom, where his sister's water had already broken. She was lying in a puddle on the linoleum floor next to the bathtub. She was pretty coolheaded; in fact, she was trying to calm her brother down during the whole process.

My partner made the woman comfortable and began assisting her. She was way too far into labor to even consider moving, so it was going to be a "field delivery"—no question about it.

Her brother was still running around, tripping over things, yelling "Oh my God," and so on. He was really, really wound up. My partner pulled me aside and told me to try to get the kid calm or occupied with something, or he was sure to hurt himself. He was a nice kid but just coming unglued before our eyes.

I thought about those old movies where somebody always yells "Boil some water!" when the baby is coming. Well, it was a bitter cold day, so I grabbed the kid and told him we were going to need warm blankets. If he could find some and put them in the dryer to warm them up, it would be a huge help.

He nodded his head like it was on a spring and shot off somewhere else in the house on his blanket mission. I went back into the bathroom to see if I was needed, and things were progressing very fast. The baby would be out any minute.

I located the laundry room to check on the nervous kid, and he's crouched in front of the dryer, telling it to hurry up, like some guy at a racetrack watching his horse run. It was doubly funny, because it was a top-loading, all-metal dryer. So the kid was doing an X-ray vision thing, willing that dryer with his mind to spin faster and hotter.

The sister had a beautiful baby right there at home. Before we headed for the hospital, we wrapped them both—in nice warm blankets.

11

Under the Checkered Flag

Fill it up with high-test. And don't count on a police escort.

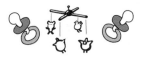

RUNNING ON EMPTY

Peter Zbytniewski is a building executive from Merrick, New York. The father of Eddie, Billy and Valerie, he now makes sure to always have a full tank of gas.

Lorraine wasn't due for another two weeks. So on this Saturday morning in May 1980, I was counting on really putting my back into doing nothing as hard as I possibly could. Maybe a little *Soul Train* (who would be the *Soul Train Scramble*–the Commodores? the O'Jays?). Maybe some wrestling or a nice, moronic gladiator movie, starring Machieste, the well-oiled, badly dubbed strong man.

I sprawled on the couch in front of the Trinitron, propped up on my left elbow. We were living in Floral Park then, in the upper level of an old house. I could see Lorraine's shadow emerge from behind the foggy glass of the shower and begin to towel off.

The Soul Train dancers were forming a gauntlet, with each kid stepping down the middle showing their moves–the best part of the show. Don Cornelius looked as cadaverous as ever.

Then I heard, "Peter? Peter, I think it's coming."

To me, this was the finest ninety seconds in all of television, but I grabbed the remote and pressed the off button like it would defuse an atom bomb. I ran into the bathroom, and Lorraine certainly didn't look like she was kidding.

"You sure? I thought you had another two weeks."

"I'm sure," she said, shooting me the hey-stupid-don't-doubt-me look. "Let's go now."

I couldn't believe it. We hadn't packed a bag. Hadn't done the pre-sign-in stuff at the hospital, hadn't even finished decorating the extra bedroom that was to be a nursery.

Lorraine threw on some clothes. I grabbed the car keys and my wallet. We walked down the stairs to the street and my trusty 1970 two-door Chrysler Newport. The thing was as long as a coal barge, handled about the same and should have come equipped with a tanker-trailer full of Sunoco 260–it got gallons to the mile.

I opened the door for Lorraine and helped her inside. Then I ran the quarter mile 'round the hood and slid behind the wheel. It turned over with that *che-che-che-che-cheeowww*–the universal song of Chrysler starters regardless of model or year. As we swung into the street, a flash of red caught my eye. It was the idiot light on the dashboard–the one that says, "Hey, bozo, you're almost out of gas."

My eyes darted right to see if Lorraine noticed, but by now she was well into labor squirms. Do I stop and pump a couple of gallons into this thing or try to make it the ten or fifteen miles to the hospital?

"Oooowwww!" Lorraine's cry made up my mind. Added to that was the usual Saturday-morning traffic. Everyone seemed to be driving like that geezer from those Pepperidge Farm commercials, just kerploppin along behind a swaybacked dray. I started to weave in and out of traffic, desperate to make the entrance ramp for the Long Island Expressway.

What was I thinking? All sorts of thoughts, one more imbecilic than the last. Glad this thing has vinyl seats in case her water breaks. Why doesn't that moron move right so I can pass? How many keys are on my key ring? Whatever happened to Cousin Brucie? Where the hell is the exit for North Shore Hospital?

"Peterrrrr! Hurry!"

Lorraine was standing up in the car! *Standing!* She had her feet on the fire wall, had locked her knees and straightened her back like a plank.

After weaving through the expressway like a madman, I hit the side streets and started blowing stop signs and red lights. I wanted to laugh. Was I Hackman in *The French Connection*? McQueen in *Bullitt*? Would my Andretti-like performance be cut short by the sickening sound of thirsty cylinders and a four-barrel carb mixing air with high-test vapor as my gold-flecked land barge rolled to a slow stop, miles from the hospital?

I kept driving, praying. *When did I last fill this thing? What did I fill it with? Does that Shell Platformate crap actually work?* Lorraine was taking those short little breaths that precede pushing. After driving like a maniac, why hadn't I picked up a motorcycle cop, who would run interference for us, just like in the movies?

At last, the hospital came into view. The emergency entrance was around back. I thought, Screw it, we might not make it, so I headed straight for the front door and drove right up on the sidewalk. I'd made it! And I could do any goddamn thing I wanted! I left the keys in and the engine running. Then I sprinted to the woman at the front desk and gave her the situation. Instantly, someone had Lorraine in a wheelchair headed for the labor room while they had me signing forms until my hand hurt. Then some guy came by and said, "You better get up there or you're gonna miss it."

I dropped the pen and ran for an elevator. As I got off, somebody held out a scrub outfit by the arms. I poked my mitts through and walked into the room just as little Eddie slipped into the world. It was beautiful.

About an hour later, somebody found us in our room and the guy handed me the keys to the car. I'd forgotten all about it!

After a while, when Lorraine seemed settled in and my eyes

were hurting from staring at Eddie through the nursery window, I headed out to the parking lot to drive home, wash up and recharge. I scanned the lot and saw the swept-back roof line of the Newport. I opened the door and turned the key. *Che-che-che-che-che-che-che-che.* The last *cheeowww* wasn't coming. It was out of gas.

PLEASE, GOD, SHOW ME A SIGN!

There are moments when Jenny Belushi's delivery could be a scene from one of her husband's movies. Here's Jim Belushi's version of the story:

 $\mathcal{W}$ hen Jenny went into labor at about ten at night, we were very calm. Jenny had her bags packed. We had even taken some trial runs to Cedars-Sinai. We were all set. Or so we thought.

First we took a long walk around the neighborhood, which is actually recommended during the early stages of labor. We just walked and talked in the darkness; and people who saw us would never have guessed that Jenny was about to give birth. She was extremely calm.

Around 4 A.M., the contractions started getting rough. Jenny was in pain, so we called the doctor, who told us to get to the hospital. We jumped into the car and were on our way.

We'd done the run to the hospital, but at four in the morning everything looks different. I was completely confused. I didn't want to tell Jenny, but I had no idea where the hell I was going. I tried to act confident, but I drove into all the wrong places at the hospital. The lots looked the same. I kept hoping I'd see a sign for the maternity ward, but I was lost. It was like being in a maze with no way out. Cedars-Sinai is a huge complex and it's so confusing. One entrance was closed. Another was for the outpatient section or something. I could tell my wife was getting frustrated with me.

I turned the music up really loud to distract her. Of course it didn't fool Jenny. To make matters worse, she was having serious contractions. "Will you please get me to the hospital!" she yelled. I started praying for a sign.

Finally I turned into a lot—the right one—pretending like this was what I had intended all along. Jenny didn't buy it, but she had other things on her mind. Her contractions were really intense at that point. This baby was on its way.

One of the best parts about the experience was that my eighteen-year-old son, Robert, was in there with us. He actually helped with the delivery, although he and I were complete idiots. We forgot how to count!

"One . . . two . . . three . . . four . . . five . . . seven . . ."

We skipped six at the same time! It was weird. Like father, like son, I guess. Despite the pain, Jenny wasn't missing anything. "You guys skipped six. What do I do now?" We laughed like hell and started all over. This time she got a full "ten count."

Toward the end of her labor, Jenny had an epidural. I'd watch the monitor and see her contractions. Even though she had no idea what was coming, I could tell when a killer contraction was on its way. But she would just smile and look at my expression and say, "Oh, that must have been a good one." She had no idea. Those contractions should have notched a 6.8 on the seismograph at Cal Tech.

When Jamison Bess was born on July 28, 1999, it was one of the most beautiful moments of my life. And to have my son in the room was incredible. He was the third person to hold my daughter. This was such a great moment for my family.

Even through the pain, my wife said that the day was like a big party. Everyone we knew was waiting outside the delivery room. Jenny kept repeating that it was the best day of her life. She had a great time. It was all worth it. Every time I look at my baby daughter, life gets better and better.

There were a lot of miracles that happened that day.

THE BOY OF SUMMER

What's the best time to have a baby? Living in the Northeast, one would assume that a warm summer evening would certainly be preferable to navigating icy winter roads. Of course, that's what one would assume— but in childbirth, all bets are off. Jeff Moorehouse, a publishing executive who now lives in Palos Verdes, California, recounts the story of his second child, Jimmy, who came along, as we all do, on his terms.

$\mathcal{M}$y second child was due any day—actually, any minute, as he was a week late. We were living back in New Jersey then. It was a hot, sticky June night and I was playing softball—center field—with the Summit, New Jersey, Men's Softball League.

Suddenly, I heard a horn blowing and saw my car coming toward the field at warp speed with my three-year-old daughter, Lauren, hanging out of the passenger window, screaming, "THE WATER JUST BROKE! THE BABY'S COMING!" My wife was at the wheel. I had no idea an '83 Jetta could move that fast. It looked like something from the Brickyard.

I dropped my mitt and jumped into the car, to the total chagrin of my teammates. In a flash we were at the hospital.

Since this was our second child, we weren't terribly stressed. Nor were the delivery room nurses who did a quick check and pronounced my wife dilated only to a number five. They hooked her up to the monitor and left us alone. Within five minutes, my wife said she was having major contractions and felt like she was ready to deliver—*immediately.*

"This can't be right," I said. After another five minutes, she screamed at me to get the nurse. I did and she ran in, checked Pam and pronounced her ready to deliver.

All hell broke loose. Our doctors hadn't been called and couldn't be reached. So the show began without them. The only person available was an intern who was told to get ready to help deliver his first baby. Next, an anesthesiologist arrived and told me he was deputizing me as his assistant.

Suddenly, everyone hoisted my wife up on the bed. She was encouraged to try to hold back the baby while they prepped her, but she just couldn't manage it. I stood at her side like the Statue of Liberty, holding an IV bag with the drugs.

Jimmy decided he wanted into our world, and all 10 pounds, 8 ounces just suddenly appeared.

An hour later, our doctors showed up. They, too, had been playing softball. I asked if they intended to discount the bill due to substitutions. But my request was, of course, denied.

IS THAT A BABY IN YOUR PANTS, OR ARE YOU JUST GLAD TO SEE ME?

Forty years ago, Helen from Minneapolis gave birth to a son in the most unusual place—her pants.

*M*y baby was about a week late so I went to see the doctor. He told me that nothing had changed—I hadn't dilated at all and the baby's head was still high. He said this baby would have to be induced. He scheduled it for later that week.

I woke up in the middle of the night. I'd been doing that a lot during this pregnancy. I went into the living room to work on my jigsaw puzzle, which usually helped me fall back to sleep. As I was doing my puzzle, I had one real hard, sharp pain in the middle of my back. I woke my husband up and we called the doctor, who said I better get to the hospital.

We didn't feel the need to rush—the hospital is only about a thirty-minute drive. Besides that one pain in my back, I hadn't shown any signs at all. My doctor didn't think I'd go into labor for days. But as I was walking to the car, my water broke and I went into full labor. I'd had four kids already, so I thought I knew the routine. I figured I still had a few more hours before this baby would show up.

But as we sped through town in our Rambler, I realized this birth would be different. I said to my husband, "This baby's coming." The contractions were so strong and the baby was really pushing. On the way, we passed a hospital for unwed mothers and my husband said, "Well, do you want to stop here?" I said, "No way! I'm a married woman!" I squeezed my legs shut.

My husband started just running through all these red lights. The funny thing was, there were cops around and they just watched us as we tore through the lights. We were still about five minutes from the hospital when I felt the baby's head go down. I was desperately trying to hold back.

Finally, we got to the hospital. My husband jumped out of the car and ran to open up the emergency entrance. The entrance was closed, so he had to hit the button to get into the garage. He was only gone for a few seconds, but during that time the baby popped out. Just like that. I didn't even try. If anything, I was holding back. I was wearing these very, very baggy maternity pants and the baby just snuggled up in those. My pants were still on. I couldn't do anything. I couldn't move. My arms were locked at my sides.

My husband ran back to the car. As he was getting into the seat, I blurted out, "Don't sit on the baby!" He looked at me, then he ran inside the hospital to get help.

I suppose the hospital was used to hysterical dads because no one took him seriously. They ignored him. He was yelling, "Help! My wife just had a baby." But people just went about their business. Finally, he saw a doctor coming down the hall. My husband yelled again, "For Pete's sake, what do you have to do to get help? There's a baby in my wife's pants!" The doctor just sort of ambled toward him and said, "Calm down. Bring your wife to admitting. Someone will check her in and get her into delivery."

My husband grabbed the doctor. "You aren't listening. It's too late for delivery. The baby's in her pants!"

Finally, they both ran to the car. I couldn't move. My whole body was frozen. The doctor somehow got the baby out of my pants, cut the cord, held him over the cement floor and whacked him on the back. It had been quite some time by then and the baby hadn't cried, so I was nervous. But after the slap on the back, the baby started howling. They ran him into the hospital

I still hadn't moved. They had to peel me out of the car. A nurse asked, "What can I do for you?" I just said, "Get me a cigarette." Thinking about it now, I know it sounds shameful, but that's all I really wanted. A cigarette.

SO, YOU DEFINITELY WON'T BE ATTENDING THE POLICEMEN'S BALL?

Mike, a film producer from Los Angeles, tells of a harrowing brush with the law while on a shoot in the Deep South.

I grew up in New York and Detroit. So I never had much experience with the mind-set of rural America. Then I spent a few weeks way below the Mason-Dixon line—so far below, in fact, that I came to regard that line not merely as a geopolitical demarcation but a portal to another dimension. Every time I flew into the rinky-dink airport, I expected to see Rod Serling dressed as a skycap, cocked eyebrow and cigarette, smirking as he welcomed me to the Twilight Zone.

We'd had weather problems, equipment problems, people problems, script problems, animal problems. On this shoot, Murphy's Law wasn't a law, it was a sentence. I'd fly back to Los Angeles when I could to be with my wife, Jackie, who was approaching full term. But then, every time I left town (if you could call it that), the shoot would go so awry that there'd be another five catastrophes, and we'd wind up further behind schedule and over budget.

Jackie wasn't from Los Angeles, either, and hadn't lived there very long, so her social circle consisted of the mailman and the kid who bagged groceries at the supermarket. When it would come time for her to deliver, I *had* to be there—not only because I didn't want to miss it for the world, but also because if I wasn't there, her only support would be from strangers.

We pressed the doctors to predict as accurately as possible when she'd deliver. But ultimately, babies come when they damn well please. We thought about having her induced, but Jackie wanted to go the natural route, and I was fully behind her decision. There will always be movie shoots from hell, but there is only one firstborn child to welcome.

As close as the doctors could determine, our baby would make her premiere on or around October 17. As the day approached, I made sure to have my bags packed and ready to go at a moment's notice. I knew all the plane schedules by heart.

Over the weeks, I actually grew accustomed to grits, Goo Goo bars and George Jones music. Southern hospitality was in full force, and the locals were very cooperative. Of course, we needed the most cooperation from the local police, and I have to say, those guys were pretty helpful. And we treated them well, too, giving them (and their families) unlimited access to craft service, photos with the stars, and as much overtime (with speedy cash payment) as they wanted.

We were just about to wrap on a stunt scene that involved ramp-jumping a car. It had taken all day because of the usual problems. The scene wasn't quite finished when I got the call from my wife—the real drama had begun.

I got into my rented car and hightailed it to the airport, about a twenty-minute drive. Did I speed? Hell yeah. The cops were my pals. I got to the airport, expecting to see the puddle jumper that was my first connection, but the runway was empty. I ran into the shack they called a terminal and asked the ticket agent (who was also the baggage handler) where my plane was. He said it was laid up in Mobile or Shreveport or something. When was the next one? "Same tahm tomorry, suh."

He checked his schedule and found that there was a flight to civilization from another tank town about sixty miles away. When did it leave? "In an ow-ah." I did the math. Sixty miles at or around the speed limit, and I could probably make it.

I hauled ass out of that airport like a stunt driver, onto the main drag, then it was pedal to the metal. Having had virtual diplomatic immunity in the locale where we were shooting, I had generally ignored speed limits. Speed limits were for tourists, and I was practically a native. Then I saw the flashing lights in my rearview. Shit!

I pulled onto the shoulder and waited. The cop was talking on the radio. And talking on the radio. And talking on the radio. Was this a cop or a talk-radio host? I kept squinting through the rearview, praying I would recognize him. No. Even with his mirrored Ray-Bans, the guy was a UFO. Which meant I was, too.

Finally, he ratcheted himself out of the car. He must have had that cruiser on some kind of load-leveling shocks, because it should have capsized from his ballast. He had to have been over four hundred pounds. By the time he walked the fifteen feet to my door, he was panting. I thought to myself, I hope fat people are jolly.

"Lah-seynce an' registrayshun," he wheezed.

No "please," I noted.

While he'd been trading doughnut recipes on the radio, I had extracted my California license from my wallet. I'd scoured my car for the rental agreement, but it was gone. Some PA had probably used it for a napkin.

"I'm sorry, Officer, but this is a rental, and I can't find the paperwork." When he saw my California license, his eyebrows arched up over his shades and his lips tightened into a slit. My mind was forming thought balloons over his head. Californ-eye-ay pinko fag thinks he can speed on mah road. Probbly one o' them Hollywood tahps. I'll slow 'im down. I'll slow 'im down gooood.

"Whut brings yuh t' these here parts?"

"I'm working on a movie over in so-and-so," I tell him. Then, trying to play the who-do-you-know card, I mentioned the sheriff with whom I'd become so palsy.

Buford, Zeke or whatever the hell his name was looked up to the sky. He couldn't tilt his head back very far. The bolster-pillow roll of fat on the back of his neck prohibited a free range of motion.

"Yeah. Well, he's theyah, an' yore heyah, an' yore commin' with me, lessin' you kin prove tuh me this shere Fawd ain't stowlen."

Jesus Christ! I'd lucked into an obese, moron cop with attitude. I recommended we call the rental company at the airport. This was before the age of the ubiquitous cell phone. I politely suggested he use his police radio.

"Yew been watchin' too many mooovies, sun. All that 'patch me through' stuff is bool-sheeyut."

"What about that?" I asked, pointing to an emergency call box down the road.

"Thass for emuhgency only."

Then I nicely told him why I was in a hurry.

"Git in the car . . . Daddy," he said as he pointed a sausage-link finger to his cop cruiser.

As I sat in the back of that cruiser staring at the chin strap of the Smoky the Bear hat buried in the fat roll on the back of his neck, I gave serious consideration to a new career—as a cop killer.

About two hours later, I was released with no apology and a ticket for speeding. The missed plane had a ripple effect. I missed the birth of my daughter, and Jackie had to go it alone.

That was over twenty years ago, and my baby girl is a junior in college. Am I still pissed? Well, I suppose I've cooled off a little. At my company, which bears my name, we get a great many calls from charities and fund-raisers. My standing instructions to my receptionist are to be very polite and request that they fax or mail more details about the cause, and we review each one and frequently make a donation. Unless it's a police charity. Those faxes and letters go straight into the garbage.

HA! YOUR SECRET IS OUT . . .

Because of traffic jams and parking problems, Marah Stets, an editor from Brooklyn, New York, had that desired natural birth. Actually, she never wavered—or did she?

At two thirty in the morning I wake up wondering, "Am I peeing or did my water break?" Still half asleep, Kevin asks me, "What's going on?" With that, there was this huge gush. In our birthing class the instructor told us that if there's no labor when your water breaks, try to go back to sleep for a while. Well, how can you sleep?

For some reason I'll never quite understand, Kevin starts programming numbers into his cell phone. He's punching in the work and home numbers of nearly everyone he knows. I don't know what possessed him, but it kept Kevin calm.

Our Lamaze teacher also told us to try to stay home as long as possible. She said once you get to the evil hospital they feed you ice chips and practically strap you down. At 4:30, I decide to take care of important business: shaving my legs. I was determined to shave them because they were so hairy. I wanted nice legs for my labor—I have no idea why. So I'm shaving, stopping every two minutes for a killer contraction. I would call out to Kevin whenever a labor pain hit. Finally, he says, "Get out of the shower." The contractions kept switching between two and three minutes apart.

At 6:30 A.M., we call the doctor, who tells us to get right in. Of course I never packed, so Kevin's tossing random stuff into my bag. I was obsessed with having warm white socks, so he packs about ten pairs. I have a bit of an issue with my feet. They're pretty ugly, plus I have this plantar wart. Well, we're nearly out the door when I become paralyzed. I sit in a rocking chair with a blanket over me. I won't budge. Kevin's talking to me and I'm not answering him. I just went into this altered state. Finally, after a half hour, I decide I'm ready to go. But I had to take my blanket with me.

It's a pretty disgusting worn-out blanket that's been washed a thousand times and has enough cat hair on it to make a few coats. It suddenly becomes my security blanket. I wrap it around me.

As we get to the car, I have this unbelievable urge to push. I grab a tree until the contraction subsides. I'm thinking, Oh my God, this baby's coming. By this time, the contractions are about two minutes apart.

When I imagined the birth, I figured I'd go into labor at home and have the baby at the hospital. I completely forgot about the car part. It never occurred to me that I'd be trapped in traffic in agonizing pain. We had to go over the Brooklyn Bridge during rush-hour traffic, so I'm arching my back the whole time trying not to push. When Kevin tells the story, he says there was hardly any traffic, but all I could see was car after car. It seemed like we were stalled for hours.

Then I have this quiet thought that I never even shared with Kevin. Throughout my pregnancy, I had been adamant about natural birth. Trapped in the car in horrible pain, all I could think about was a nice epidural. Screw the natural birth thing—the minute I get to that hospital I want a needle stuck in me!

New York City hospitals aren't the most accommodating places. You don't just pull into a big ol' lot and park your car in front of an entrance. There's absolutely no parking. I yell at Kevin to leave the car anywhere, but thankfully he didn't do that or we'd still be paying tow-truck expenses. Kevin drives the wrong way down one-way streets to find a parking garage. Finally he backs down Seventeenth Street to pull into a lot.

Next thing I know we're at the reception desk. We're pre-registered, but of course they have none of our papers. I'm kind of a reserved person, but I'm squealing like a stuck pig, "I'm pushing. I'm pushing. This baby's coming." I've got my trusty security blanket draped around me. People in the waiting room occasionally glance up from over newspapers to see who the insane woman is.

By 8 A.M., I'm in a room. Seconds later, the head crowns. Forty minutes later, the baby is halfway out and Kevin goes, "Okay, okay. What do you think?" I say very confidently, "I know it's a boy."

Mothers have these instincts, I thought. I push a few times and out plops a little girl, Marlena Claire, weighing 6 pounds, 6 ounces.

Thanks to rush-hour traffic and city parking nightmares, I never did get that epidural. So I had my natural childbirth experience. Kevin doesn't know I ever wavered. Let him think I'm a hero.

As they wheel me into recovery, I'd never felt so exhilarated in my life. Then I look down and see that my trusty blanket is covering me. Gee, is it filthy, I think.

12

You Shall Herewith Be Touched

Is there any event as heartwarming as the birth of a baby?

These could melt steel.

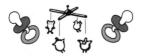

BABY . . . LOVE

This book is dedicated to moms throughout the universe. As co-author, I'd be remiss if I didn't include a worthy story about the greatest mother I know, my own.

I remember a particular St. Patrick's Day in New York, when the weather veered across Manhattan like a runaway cyclorama. Brilliant sunshine would flood the street then instantly vanish as Fifth Avenue was plunged into deep shadow. Next, a moment of snow flurries, until the blinding sun again forced shading hands to foreheads in salutes to its power.

Vendors dotted the crowd, hawking everything from gaudy, Frisbee-sized Kiss-Me-I'm-Irish buttons to stuffed toys with no more relation to the event than the hideous acid green they had been dyed the day before. I wanted to stop and look at their tacky merchandise, but Mom would sweep past them, contemptuous of their garish junk.

For several blocks we hurried along the narrow corridor between onlookers' backs and the buildings, until she found a monger with the wares she sought—fresh shamrocks floating in a bucket of ice water. She paid him a few coins, then pinned a bunch to my lapel. We worked our way into the crowd and finally stood at the wooden police barricade—she above it, me below—both with a panoramic view of the parade. We watched the procession of ruddy-kneed, high-stepping majorettes, white-gloved marching bands and sash-draped dignitaries tramp past. I could feel the percussive boom of bass drums as they echoed between the skyscrapers.

My mother, born and raised in Ireland, was fiercely proud of her heritage. She leaned low and spoke into my ear. "See, Larry? You're Irish. And this parade is because everybody loves the Irish!"

I was maybe five at the time and had little grasp of a place called Ireland or the concept of heritage. The comment might have faded into the mists of forgotten childhood memories, but I noticed a tear streaming down her cheek. I'll never know what recollection or emotion seized her at that moment, but it was doubtless quite powerful.

We had an appointment to keep. Turning our backs on the parade, we headed to a corner to cross the street, and there she grabbed my hand. Certain I could navigate any intersection solo, I defiantly wriggled my hand free from hers. She bent down and said, "Come on, Larry, hold my hand just while we cross this street. Someday when you're a big, grown-up man and I'm an old lady, I'll take your hand when you ask. I promise."

I surrendered my hand. And she kept her promise.

Were this ten or twelve years ago, she'd have written her own story and done a far better job of it than I. But over time her formidable powers with the written and spoken word have been stolen by the relentless, cruel thievery of Alzheimer's.

An abundantly gifted woman, my mother evinced extraordinary talents as a singer, artist, poet, writer and raconteur. She could have had her pick of those professions but instead chose the one that made her heart sing—motherhood. Throughout her life, her astonishing skills remained avocations, for she would never, ever rob a single moment from the work she loved best—raising her two sons.

Perhaps for her, motherhood was more of an imperative than a choice. Her obsession with babies bloomed when she was barely out of her own infancy. She would baby-sit any infant, any time, anywhere, for free. My grandfather told me her maternal fire burned so strong that he sometimes worried she'd take a baby from an unguarded pram.

She loved children, and they loved her. She could not pass a baby carriage without a peek inside and a chat with the occupant. Small kids sought her out and clung to her, sensing her love. Many a baby, after spending just a few minutes in my mother's arms, would refuse to return to its own parent. Mom was a baby magnet—she was uncanny.

When my daughter, Olivia, was born, I couldn't wait to introduce her to my mother. As soon as possible, Irene and I took Olivia to the home where my mother resides with several other Alzheimer's patients.

Always adept at keeping me on an even keel, Irene reminded me that I might be disappointed. Over the past couple of years, Mom had declined to where she could no longer speak—even smiles were very, very rare. Almost all the wires were down.

I knelt by my mother's easy chair, where she sometimes stares interminably at a spot on the carpet.

"Hi, Mommy. How are you today?"

There was no response, no reaction.

But as I placed her fat, gurgling, swaddled granddaughter in her lap, her eyes widened and burned with an awareness they'd not held in a long, long time. She took the baby in her arms, clutched her to her breast, beamed and rocked back and forth.

"Baby . . . Love," she said. Those were the first words she had uttered in well over a year.

THE BIRTHDAY MESSAGE

Christin Conklin of Eastchester, New York, didn't believe in angels until she received a very special delivery.

I've had four children and the first thing I do when I start contracting is take a shower and put on makeup. The whole bit. You've got to look your best even if you don't feel your best. I have a lot of incentive. My doctor is so cute. He's a doll. I make sure I have my makeup kit right next to me in the delivery room. Sometimes I'll even do touch-ups on the table. Despite the pain, I've got on my blush, eyeliner and lipstick. I also make a point of getting waxed every four weeks. You don't want to be hairy when you're pushing out your baby.

That's more important than anything they teach you in Lamaze. I'll tell you—all that Lamaze stuff goes out the window in the delivery room. Anthony, my husband, will say things like "Focal point. Get a focal point." I just have to laugh. What's a focal point when you'd rather be dead? With one of my sons, I said, "Okay, God, I'm ready. Take me now." I could not imagine that you could be in that much pain and still be alive.

I had three sons when I became pregnant again. I really, really wanted a girl, but I didn't want to know beforehand. I figured, If it's a boy, the minute I see him, I'll love him. But I couldn't imagine a household filled with that much testosterone. Besides, I had saved all my dolls and toys from childhood. I wanted a daughter to play with them or give me a good excuse to play with them.

It was October 25, 2000—a week before my due date. I was running around all day feeling very anxious. Toward the end of the day, I decided I needed a pedicure to relax. Plus, the last thing I wanted was to go into labor with bad toenails. What a way to turn off my cute doctor.

After the pedicure, I decided a manicure was in order. But first I had to go to the bathroom. Well, I'm in the bathroom at the

salon and I'm going and going and going. It just wasn't stopping.
I'm thinking, How could this be? I only drank half a can of soda
at four o'clock! Then it slowly dawned on me—my water must
have broken.

In all my births, I never had my water break on its own. So I
didn't know what it was like. I had been told you'd hear a pop,
but I didn't hear anything. I'm sitting there, thinking, How do I
stop this? I'm waiting and waiting, but it's still gushing out of me.
It seemed like hours had gone by, but it was only minutes. I didn't
know what to do. The door was locked, so I couldn't scream for
someone to come in and help me.

Finally, it subsided a bit. I jammed about a dozen paper towels
down my pants. Then, very slowly, I waddle out. I tell the mani-
curist, "I don't think I'll be getting my nails done today. My water
just broke." She gave me a towel and I wore it like a diaper.

I still had the little paper slippers on my feet with the paper
wrapped between each toe. I'm walking out with this towel diaper
and paper slippers on. My toenails weren't dry, so after all that
work, why smudge them?

I drove home and my husband took me to the hospital. At
7 P.M., I was only two centimeters dilated. I was having contractions every two to three minutes.

But I didn't want to have the baby yet anyway. I wanted to wait
until the next day. October 26 was my father's birthday. He had
died nearly four years earlier and I thought it would be a really
nice way to celebrate his birthday. I kept praying, Any time after
midnight.

Midnight came and went. Everyone in the room said, "Okay,
it's your dad's birthday—you can have that baby now." We're
watching the World Series. I'm doing squats. I'm moving from
side to side. The nurse gives me an enema and I didn't care.
Anything to get this baby out. About 2:30 A.M., the pain becomes
unbearable. They give me Stadol and I start hallucinating. For
some reason, all I wanted to do was go sleigh riding. I haven't
sledded since I was a kid, but it's all I can think about. Then I
blurt things out. I tell my husband I love him. Then I tell him I

want him, right then and there. Right on the delivery-room table. I shut my eyes and plead with myself to fall asleep—because God knows what I would have said or done next.

When I wake up, I'm about six centimeters. They give me an epidural. By 10, I'm nine centimeters. At 10:30, I'm nine and a half centimeters. My doctor says, "Okay, you can start pushing." After eighteen hours of labor, the baby just plops out. I only needed to push for twenty minutes.

"What do you think it is?"

Of course it's a boy. We named him Chad because Chad is an English saint and the name means one of four brothers. My father's name was Frank, so Chad's middle name is Frank Michael after my father and his twin brother.

Chad Frank Michael is my only child who never met his grandfather. But then I thought about it and decided that my dad sent this baby to me on his birthday as a message. He wanted me to know that he had seen his grandson. I could almost hear him saying, "Don't worry, honey, you're not getting your daughter."

MONKEY SOUNDS

Peggy Noonan, the former speechwriter for Ronald Reagan, is an author of several best-selling books and a frequent contributor to *The Wall Street Journal, The New York Times* and others. She often appears on television, offering her perspective of the political scene.

She had these touching recollections about her son's birth.

*W*hen I think of the birth of my son, I first recall the last few days prior to his arrival. I had looked at one of those calendars that show which famous people were born on each day. For June 12, they had Anne Frank, who was such an important person to me when I was a child, and with whom I so identified, as many children of my generation did. I thought, How beautiful if my son were born on the birth date of someone I care so much about. So I hoped.

On June 11, I had a checkup and my blood pressure was too high, so the doctor said, "We're inducing—get to the hospital." It was about noon. I got to the hospital, labor was induced, my son was born healthy and I was fine. While I was holding him for the first time I said, "What time was he born?" and someone said, "11:17 P.M., June 11." I thought, Oh. And then I realized: In Europe, where Anne lived, it is dawn on the twelfth, and someone is thinking of her now and marking this day. I will always feel that my son was born on Anne Frank's birthday, which still pleases me.

I went through labor in the cardiac unit of intensive care because my doctors suspected I had a condition called peripartum cardiomyopathy. And if you have that condition, you might have a heart attack after giving birth. I had had heart problems during the pregnancy, serious enough to require absolute bed rest the last few months. But I didn't think I had the condition everyone feared I had. Anyway, as my son was born the cardiologist was frantically monitoring my heart, and a team was standing by for my attack, and they almost lost track of the fact that a baby was being born. So it was an odd ambiance in the delivery room. (I didn't have the heart attack.)

Then I remained in the cardiac intensive care unit rather than in a maternity ward. And I had nurses who didn't know what to do with a woman who'd just had a baby! Since it was my first I didn't know what to ask for. But it all turned out fine and in a few days I was in the maternity ward. But I realized: When you have a baby you want to be surrounded by people who have just had a baby, and you also want to be surrounded by people who treat women who have just had a baby.

I was almost taken aback—maybe that's not the way to say it, but certainly I was delighted and grateful—at how much I loved my child. It was immediate. I had always wondered if you learn to love a child or if it just happens at some point, but I realized I loved him before I held him.

My favorite memory of life is nursing him at home in a big sun-filled room when he was a few months old. We would make cooing and crooning sounds at each other. Around that time there was a special on PBS about monkeys and their babies. The monkeys made these funny little sounds at their babies and I found it enchanting. I made these soft sounds at my son, and in time he made them back. He's a teenager now, but to this day when we hug we unconsciously make the monkey sound and then hear it and start to laugh.

It is a matter of amusement and embarrassment to me that I make the monkey sound whenever I hug anyone I love. They are sometimes surprised—but no one has ever complained, and I think they now know it's what I do.

IN ALL THINGS, REJOICE

Lisa Whelchel spent nine years playing the stuck-up Blair on the television sitcom *The Facts of Life*. These days, the devout Christian is busy homeschooling Haven, Tucker and Clancy, her children with husband Steven Cauble, a pastor. When daughter Haven was born, Lisa, who lives in Santa Clarita, California, says she witnessed a miracle.

Tucker, my first child, was upside down in the womb, so I had to schedule a C-section and was very disappointed—I couldn't believe it. We had just finished our Lamaze classes and I had broken the hospital record in the "sniff-sniff, shee-shee, hold ten, long blow" event. I was ready to go for the gold, but I didn't even qualify for the finals.

So from the moment the little stick turned blue indicating my second pregnancy, I was determined to have this baby "like a real woman." I had many conversations with my doctor—he going about his OB/GYN examining duties, I talking as if we were merely chatting over a cup of tea. He assured me that I would be able to have a V-BAC this time. I was relieved, thinking this meant lying on my back with my legs in the V position, which is what I wanted the first time. He informed me V-BAC stood for "Vaginal Birth After Cesarean." Even better!

I was reading in bed when my water broke at 8:30 P.M., and already my contractions were coming pretty furiously. By the time we got to the hospital I was ready for the epidural. I practically asked the parking attendant to give it to me, but he wouldn't. Once inside, I changed into something a little more comfortable, my hospital lingerie with the easy-open back. The nurse untied the little string and I finally felt the pain to end all pain—the blessed epidural. I was home free! I had made it through the hard part!

My doctor arrived and I assumed our traditional conversation pose while he checked my progress. He assured me that everything was going fine and that it would be time to push soon.

Steve and I relaxed and went back to watching *The Tonight Show*. The doctor joined me again a few minutes later to check all my digital hookups. Then he leaned over and said something to the attending nurse. She went scurrying out.

Pandemonium broke out in the labor room and he informed me that the baby's heartbeat was dangerously erratic and he was going to have to perform an emergency C-section. I was crushed. My dream was not going to come true. I couldn't believe I had made it through the hardest part and I still was not going to get to experience a traditional childbirth. As they were wheeling me down to the operating room, I heard the Lord whisper to me, "Rejoice in all things." I begrudgingly uttered through my clenched teeth, "Okay, Lord, thank You that I'm having this C-section. I will praise You in all things and I will rejoice in You."

As the doctor made the incision, I saw the look on his face. He motioned Steve over to take a picture of my stomach. There was a gaping hole just beneath the first layer of skin. My previous C-section scar had ruptured six of the seven sewn layers to expose a small window. In an instant I realized that had I delivered my daughter Haven the way I had wanted to, we would not have known about the rupture until later and after much internal bleeding. And that's not even the primary miracle in this story.

To my and my doctor's shock, in my birth canal I was harboring the often-fatal blood disease Group B streptococcus. Had Haven been born vaginally, she would have ingested the bacteria on her way out. Thankfully, my baby never passed through the canal. If she had, she could have died. But it's no mystery why she survived. Haven was born at 2:46 A.M. on September 26, 1991, weighing 7 pounds, 3 ounces. And again I say, "Rejoice." Sometimes the Lord says "No" to our dreams in order to birth something healthier in our lives.

AN UNEXPECTED GIFT

Dynasty, The Love Boat, Fantasy Island, Melrose Place, Beverly Hills 90210, Charmed—the list is endless. Aaron Spelling is, without question, the most successful television producer ever. He's also a devoted family man. His two children, Randy and Tori, are his pride and joy.

Tori hit her cue precisely—she was born on time and without any difficulty. Little Randy was born on October 9, 1978, quite a bit ahead of schedule. And when he came into the world, he weighed only two and a half pounds. Then he shrank to just two pounds.

Of course we had to keep him at the hospital, and I would visit him in the morning before I went to the studio. Candy, my wife, would stay at the hospital all day. Then I'd run back constantly to look in on them both. This was at Cedars-Sinai, and they had just been equipped with some new lights that shone down into the crib. These lights were like magic—all the doctors marveled at them and told me that these lights were the major reason why Randy was alive and starting to thrive. They were called Incubator Blue Lights.

Back then, Leonard Goldenson owned ABC Television. We did a lot of business together and were very, very good friends. Leonard called from New York right after Randy was born and said he wanted to fly in to see Randy. So I said sure, that would be great, and he arrived the next day. I picked him up at his hotel and then we drove over to Cedars-Sinai. We had to put on gowns and gloves and masks because these infants were all so fragile.

As we stood over Randy, I very excitedly told Leonard that these Incubator Blue Lights were some new invention that had actually saved my son's life. I was so thrilled by the miracle of the technology. Though I couldn't see Leonard's smile beneath the mask, his eyes were absolutely beaming—actually tearing—with joy. He said, "You don't know what this means to me." Perplexed, I asked him what. He then told me he had put up the money to research and develop those Incubator Blue Lights.

Now what are the chances of that happening? I just stood there crying like a baby. I must have hugged him sixteen times.

After a while, I drove him back to his hotel. He checked his watch and said, "Hey, I can still make it out to the airport." I couldn't believe my ears. He flew in that morning to see my son and he was flying back that night—a grueling feat for anyone, and he was no kid at the time.

When we brought Randy home, Tori was attached to him until he could walk, then they fought all the time. What thrills me most is that they are the best friends you could imagine two people could possibly be. Candy and I get goosebumps every time we see them together.

Funny Things Said in Childbirth

Repeat these actual quotations at your next birthing experience. You'll raise eyebrows. You'll get laughs. You'll get slapped.

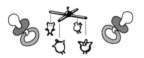

1. "Make it stop for a while. I need my sleep."

2. "I changed my mind."

3. A woman jumped off the bed, leaped into the nurse's arms, crossed her legs and said, "I can't do this anymore. I'm gonna hold it in till I'm good and ready."

4. One husband tried to sneak out to have a cigarette break. The wife said, "You get your fucking ass back in here. You were there in the beginning. You're going to suffer with me right through to the end."

5. A woman grabbed a nurse by the front of her shirt, pulled her nose-to-nose and screamed, "It's coming out the wrong hole!"

6. "What time will this baby be born?"

7. "Can I get an epidural for my sympathy pains?"
   —a husband to a nurse

8. "Can you stitch my wife to make her tighter?"

9. "Get it out right now. I don't care how. Just pull it out now. Open me up if you have to."

10. "I've got to poop. It's not the baby's head—I'm pooping. I know the difference."

11. "I really think I'm going to split in half."

12. "Is it possible for my ass to fall off?"

13. "That wasn't so bad, huh? We'll have another one soon."
    —*husband to wife after twenty hours of labor*

14. "That baby can't be mine—no one has a smushed-up face in my family."
    —*husband to wife*

15. "Is that baby going to get better-looking?"
    —*husband to no one in particular*

16. "That's not its full size? Is it?"
    —*a dad to the doctor about his newborn's penis*

17. "Stitch me up like a virgin, please."

18. "It's a baby!"

19. "What's the matter with his penis?"
    —*father observing newborn daughter*

20. "I have sinned, and now I am in hell!"
    —*mother in labor*

21. "I AM visualizing a spot on the ceiling—and it looks like a stretching vagina!"
    —*mother in labor*

22. "Do you have the tools there to give him a vasectomy?"
    —*mom to doctor as her episiotomy is being sutured*

23. "He's got a hard-on. Wonder what's turning him on?"
    —*new dad on observing son's erection*

24. "Look, honey, he's better hung than you are."
    —*mom to dad*

25. "It's got your nose—and your old boyfriend's eyes."
    —*husband to wife*

26. "Let's make a wish!"
    —*husband to nurse while they each hold one of Mom's legs as she prepares to push*

27. "Just ignore him. He does that all the time."
    —*wife about husband who passed out during delivery*

28. "I'LL NEVER HAVE SEX WITH YOU AGAIN!"

14

In a League of Their Own

Some stories defy categorization.

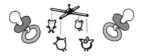

EXTRATERRESTRIALS AND TORNADOES

In 1992, Erin Brockovich was a struggling, divorced mother of three working at a law firm for $800 a month. Then she discovered that a utility company was contaminating a town's water supply. After helping win one of the largest class-action suits in history, the Los Angeles resident became the subject of the eponymous blockbuster movie starring Julia Roberts. But even if Erin hadn't found fame through her courageous legal battle, it would have found her, because she's such an extraordinary personality. Though quite proud of the film, she's quick to point out that it never covered the most important part of her life—the births of her three kids, Matthew, Katie and Elizabeth.

I was at the movies watching *E.T.* when I suddenly felt very strange. But it had nothing to do with getting emotional over that little extraterrestrial. My back ached and I felt queasy. Even though I'd never had a baby before, I could just tell it was the beginning of labor.

I was living in Lawrence, Kansas, and the town was under a tornado watch. There was thunder and torrential rain. I went straight home, sat on the toilet and lost my mucus plug. I had really bad diarrhea, but that had nothing to do with labor pains. I always get diarrhea when there's the impending danger of a serious storm. And I'm always on the toilet when there's a tornado warning. Actually, I wasn't even nervous about going into labor. I barely thought about it because I was so petrified of the tornado. Childbirth seemed like a piece of cake next to a tornado.

My mom drove me to the hospital because my husband was working in Kansas City. With the storm it took him over an hour to get to the hospital. When they checked me in, I was only one centimeter dilated, but the contractions were strong and consistent. In four hours, I was nine centimeters dilated.

I went through Lamaze, but all along I thought, This is bullshit. When I'm in pain don't ask me to stare at some focal point and don't tell me how to breathe. I'll throw all that crap right out the window. If I'm going to yell, I'll yell. Picturing a white puffy cloud floating by isn't going to stop me from screaming my lungs out.

I guess I was doing just that when a nurse came in and glared at me. "It can't be that bad," she said. I was ready to chop off her head. "You're fucking kidding me, right? How the hell would you know what *my* pain is like?"

Everyone has a different threshold for pain. My mother gets root canals with no painkillers, but I'm a baby when it comes to pain. So many people get set on having natural childbirth, but if it's something you don't completely want to do, I think it's fine to have an epidural.

I was really screaming—I wanted this baby out. But the head wasn't showing. The doctor who examined me was the same doctor who had delivered me twenty-three years earlier. He said, "There's no head engaged because that's the butt."

That was scary. They immediately rushed me for a C-section. I was knocked out for it and when I woke up there was my beautiful son, Matthew. He was 7 pounds, 14 ounces. I found out later that he had been born blue with the umbilical cord wrapped around his neck. It could have been a horrible situation, but I didn't even think about it at the time. I had this little healthy baby in my arms.

I like to say I was fortunate enough to have three C-sections, so I only really had pain for the first birth. Matt was only five months old when I became pregnant with Katie. I went to the doctor because I thought I had the flu. Then he called me to say, "Guess what? The rabbit died." I said, "How can that be? I don't even remember the last time I had sex. This has to be another Immaculate Conception." Katie's and Elizabeth's births were nice and easy.

But to tell you the truth, no one remembers the pain. Once that beautiful baby is in your arms, you forget all about the pain. There's nothing but joy. I can remember the sting of a shot more than the pain of childbirth or the pain of recovering from C-sections.

Since the movie *Erin Brockovich* came out, I've been doing a lot of motivational speaking and I realized that a lot of what I say could be applied to childbirth. This is my advice:

1. If the pain's gonna get you, you shouldn't have gotten pregnant.

2. You're going to be scared. It will hurt. But tough shit. It's going to happen. You've got to stick it out. Accept it. Don't fight it because it's inevitable.

3. Remember, the outcome will be great.

4. This is as easy as it gets. If you think the birth's scary, wait until you have teenagers. Now that's scary. They're yours forever.

5. Don't listen to the horror stories. Remember, opinions are like assholes: Everyone's got one.

6. Eat a lot. It's about losing weight after.

I finally went back and saw *E.T.* in its entirety. I've seen it many times since Matt was born in 1983. Funny thing, for a long time that was his favorite movie. Now he's eighteen and I have no idea what his favorite movie is.

The other day when I was at a restaurant, I saw this cute guy in jeans and thought, "Hmmmm, he's a babe." Then I realized it was my son. It feels like it was just yesterday when I was holding him in my arms for the first time.

ONE, NO . . . MAKE THAT TWO FOR THE ROAD

Midge Zimmerli, who owns a Chicago-based landscaping company, anesthetized herself for the birth of her third son, Shawn.

Since this was baby number three, I had achieved a certain level of confidence. After all, the first two deliveries had been pretty smooth.

At the time we were living in Latham, New York, which is near Albany. It was July 8, 1964, one of the hottest, muggiest days I can recall. Barbara, my friend from across the street, came by to gab and we both agreed that a cold beer would be just fabulous. "I think I have one in my fridge," Barbara offered. I hadn't even had a cup of coffee during my pregnancy, never mind a beer. But I was so close to delivery I knew it wasn't going to hurt my baby.

Barbara shot through the screen door and across the lawn. Locusts were buzzing, and the humidity was so high it sort of stung your skin. In a flash, Barbara was coming back across the street carrying one of those big quart bottles of beer, the kind construction workers use to wash down their submarine sandwiches.

We flopped under a tree and pried the cap off. It was icy cold and the first splash was pure thirst-quenching ambrosia. The second glass was about as good as the first and pretty soon that bottle was dead empty. Well, that beer didn't affect the weather one bit, so we both decided to see if another bottle might bring in a cold front.

It was so hot, we didn't even realize we'd caught a buzz. That's about when my contractions began. For a while, I ignored them.

Before my second son, Craig, had been born, I had a false labor, so I wasn't about to be the girl who cried wolf again.

When the contractions reached about fifteen minutes apart, I figured it was pretty real. So I phoned my husband, and he raced home from work. By then, Barbara had sounded the general alarm in the neighborhood. When Dick pulled up, there was a little crowd on the front lawn.

My overnight bag had been packed for days, so I grabbed it, got in the car and we took off, as all these housewives waved us away. It was so kooky, like a bon voyage for a couple of newlyweds.

I don't recall if the car had air-conditioning or if it was broken, but it was pretty hot in that car. On the way to the hospital, we passed a little neighborhood watering hole.

"I've gotta have a beer," I announced.

"What?"

"It's hot. I'm thirsty; and they're sure not going to give me one at the hospital, so pull over, I'm getting a beer."

Dick pulled up in front. I ran inside, ordered a short one and gulped it down. The bartender never even took his eye off the television. I ran back to the car. Even though it was just a little one, it must have been pretty powerful, because that's about when everything got really, really funny.

At the hospital, I thought everything was a joke, especially when the doctor asked me if I'd had a drink.

"Of course I have!"

Then he advised me that in that case, there'd be no anesthetic.

"No problem. I doubt I'll feel much pain, ha ha ha ha!"

I must have been pretty funny, because everyone in that room was howling through my entire labor.

Well, those beers did the trick. I had Shawn just as easy as can be. He must have been the easiest delivery in history because I was so relaxed and laughing.

I'm sure people will read this and eyebrows will lift. But really, I'm inclined to think a couple of beers were as effective, and likely safer, than an epidural, or whatever intravenous drug they offered in those days.

GO AHEAD, NAME MY KID

Clint and Dina Ruiz Eastwood met in 1993, when the then news anchor in Salinas, California, interviewed the actor/director just after his Western, *Unforgiven*, had won four Oscars. The reporter and Dirty Harry fell in love and married, and in 1996 became parents. As Dina tells it, the story of how their daughter was named is pure Hollywood.

Clint was in Los Angeles and I was at our home in Carmel, missing him. So I decided to visit my husband. I wasn't due until later in December–I figured a little trip would be a nice distraction. Not that my pregnancy was horrible; although I was really sick and needed to be hooked to an IV for the first six weeks, the rest of my pregnancy was a breeze. I worked, hit a lot of golf balls and never got weird or winded toward the end.

I got to Los Angeles, saw Clint and then decided to spend the afternoon Christmas shopping with a friend. I hadn't bought any Christmas presents yet, so I was all excited. As I grabbed my purse, I suddenly remembered that I had missed my weekly doctor's appointment. My friend called her doctor and he was able to squeeze me in.

As he examined me, he said, "Has this baby moved today?" I thought about it and said, "Well, yes. Just a little while ago." He did some tests and determined that the baby was in trouble. There was something wrong with my placenta. He said, "You're going to have to be induced." I was in shock. "What are you talking about? I'm going Christmas shopping."

I checked into the hospital, but I was annoyed. I didn't really understand what was going on. I was sprawled out on a couch reading a magazine when a nurse walked in and asked, "Who's Dina?"

I say, "Me."

"Get your ass in the gown. You're the patient," she says. She was this tough but sweet New Yorker type.

"You don't understand. I'm not ready to have this baby."
They didn't agree. They induced me with Pitocin, but the baby still wouldn't come. Hours and hours went by.

Clint and I watched some television. During the height of my labor, we watched Jay Leno. I just kept laughing and laughing because I was so high on something. My labor was never awful.

I eventually opted for an epidural. They gave me one and I was still up and about. At one point, I was in the bathroom and a nurse came in the room, freaked out and started checking under the bed. She thought I'd passed out and slid under the bed. They told me that they'd never seen anybody walking around after getting an epidural. It was all pretty goofy.

When it was time for me to push, Clint was at our L.A. home napping. They told me that if I wanted my husband there for the birth, I'd better not sneeze. Well, Clint drove eighty miles an hour and was back at the hospital in a few minutes. Once he was there, the doctor said, "Okay." I swear I barely had to push. She was out in about two minutes. I'd been in labor for twenty-four hours.

Our daughter was born at noon on December 12, 1996, weighing 8 pounds, 4 ounces. Clint cut the cord. He's not squeamish at all. He's actually into all that medical stuff—he's fascinated with medicine. He's an honorary M.D. in my book. If he hadn't been an actor, he would have made a great doctor.

All along we thought we were having a boy. So when this girl came out, we didn't know what to call her. We'd thought about Olivia and Alana but couldn't make up our minds.

Because we didn't want to be harassed by the tabloids, I'd checked into the hospital as Dina Morgan, which is my mother's maiden name. When we were discharged the next day, we had to fill out forms with the baby's name on it. I asked what the rule was on naming a baby after leaving the hospital. They told me we'd both have to come back to the hospital within the next ten days and fill out forms. Well, Clint and I were ready to get back to Carmel—I couldn't imagine trekking to Los Angeles with a newborn.

Clint said, "Wait a minute. We're going to name this baby right now."

At the same time, we looked down at the little Plexiglas bassinet where our daughter was sleeping. On the side it said "Baby Morgan." We thought for a moment and agreed—Morgan would be our daughter's name. We'd never even considered it before, but Morgan made complete sense. Since it's my mom's maiden name, it is all the more special to me. So in some strange way I have the tabloids to thank for my daughter's name.

HEY, DOC, WHILE YOU'RE OUT, GET YOURSELF A SEX CHANGE

Judy, a nurse from Westchester County, New York, thought she'd seen it all. That was, until she met Omed and Ishla. (Some names have been changed for the usual reasons.)

There was a blizzard raging when Omed and Ishla entered the delivery room at four in the morning. Even though Ishla was already ten centimeters dilated, the couple seemed extremely calm—almost too calm for first-time parents.

The husband shook my hand. "I am Omed and this is my wife, Ishla. She is in quite a bit of pain but does not want drugs of any kind."

Ishla squeezed out a half smile. She was in her early twenties and very pretty. Omed was in his mid-thirties. They were from somewhere in the Middle East but living in White Plains, New York, where Omed was a Web designer.

Since Ishla was already dilated, I called their doctor. Due to the storm, the roads were blocked and she was stranded in Mount Kisco, which was about ten miles from the hospital. I knew this baby might come any minute so I paged Dr. Leslie Armstrong, her partner. Then I informed the couple.

Omed was wiping Ishla's face with a wet compress. When I

told him that his doctor wouldn't make it in time, Omed leapt from his chair.

"This cannot be happening! I demand Ishla's doctor. Doesn't the hospital provide helicopters for emergencies like this?"

Omed was right in my face and his spit flew as he spoke. I stepped back and politely explained that Dr. *Leslie* Armstrong was extremely capable of delivering their baby. Ishla smiled at him and Omed appeared to relax.

"This baby is ready to come out. Let's start pushing," I said.

As if on cue, Dr. Armstrong threw open the door.

"Okay, folks, let's get this baby out," he barked. Then he stretched out his hand to Omed. "I'm Dr. . . ."

Omed's eyes bugged out of their sockets. "Get out of here right now!"

Dr. Armstrong's mouth dropped. He looked at me. I shrugged my shoulders.

"The last time I checked, I was the doctor. This is my delivery room."

"You are very mistaken. We are waiting for a Dr. Leslie."

"I am Dr. Leslie Armstrong."

Omed sneered. "Leslie is a woman's name."

Dr. Armstrong laughed. "I agree. I don't know what my mother was thinking."

But Omed wasn't amused. His eyes narrowed as he studied the doctor. "I won't have a perverted American man touching my wife."

Dr. Armstrong smiled. "I assure you, I've delivered hundreds of babies—none telekinetically."

The baby's hairy little head was showing. It would only be a few minutes before this child plopped into the world.

"Keep pushing. Come on, Ishla," I said.

"Stop pushing! You will not continue with this man in here! I forbid it."

Ishla was in tears. She grunted. "I can't stop pushing! It's pushing on its own."

"Then push it back." Omed spoke through clenched teeth.

Dr. Armstrong took a few steps toward Ishla.

"Cover her up," Omed yelled at me. Then he turned toward the doctor. "I've told you before, do not get any closer to my wife!"

This was hardly a time for modesty—the baby's head was sticking out. Ishla looked at me, her black eyes full of terror.

I tried the best I could to block out the lunacy. I counted to ten with her. I instructed her to push. To exhale. I could tell Ishla wasn't giving it her all. She was obeying her husband and holding back.

I concentrated on Ishla. Behind me I heard the doctor pleading with Omed. "Just let me catch the baby. I won't even look at your wife."

Through Ishla's screams, I heard Omed saying something about sick American men with their pornography. Their Internet sites. Their magazines. I bit my cheeks to stop from smiling.

The baby was nearly out. I turned toward the doctor. Omed stood in front of him like a point guard blocking a shot. It was a dance. The doctor moved, Omed moved with outstretched arms. I turned back to Ishla. The doctor was suddenly gone.

"You may have this baby now," Omed said. "We don't need any doctor."

Which is how I've always felt. I'm there from the beginning, listening to the complaints. Cleaning the blood, the vomit and, yes, the poop. My ears ring for days from the screams. The curses. The fights. Then, five minutes before the birth, the doctor shows up and takes all the glory. The big hero catches the baby, while the nurse fades into the background.

"Come on, push!"

When the baby slid out, I caught it. Easy.

"It's a girl," I said as the baby starting howling.

A few seconds later, Dr. Armstrong was back in the room. As the doctor grabbed the infant from me, Omed wiped tears from his eyes and hugged his wife.

I looked at this beautiful baby girl and thought, Poor Daddy. Wait until she starts dating those perverted American boys.

WELL, HE DID GET YOU PREGNANT . . . DIDN'T HE?

Marie O'Hara lives in Quincy, Massachusetts, and has three children. She also has a few issues with her husband and technology.

*L*et me start off by saying that my husband, Ron, should be living in Amish country because he can't operate anything more complicated than a paper clip. You have no idea—he demolishes any kind of device or appliance. We go through about two VCRs every year. He broke my washing machine because he turned the knob the wrong way. One of our cars needed an engine overhaul because he never noticed that it takes premium, not regular, gas. Oh, and how about an oil change at 18,000 miles? Tire rotation? What's that?

I know it sounds like role reversal. Usually the man is more mechanically inclined. Don't get me wrong—he's male in every other way. But if it clicks, whirs, has batteries or a motor, forget it.

What he doesn't wreck by ignorance he'll destroy by clumsiness. He dropped his electric shaver into a sink full of water. Ditto my hair dryer. The blender got bogged down when he was making thick shakes, so he stuck a spoon in—deep. What a sound that made when it hit those spinning blades!

The house looks like a graffiti gang got in there. I tape instruction notes to everything. NO METAL IN THE MICROWAVE! QUIT APPLICATIONS BEFORE SHUTTING DOWN COMPUTER! DON'T FORGET TO UNPLUG COFFEE MACHINE! They don't do any good. For the first few days he notices them, then they just blend in with the wallpaper. I swear, the local repairmen are counting on us to put their kids through college.

Even when he's trying to be helpful, it backfires. On that brand-new car, he cleaned the plastic instrument panel with glass cleaner. So now there's permanent fog over all the gauges. I have to guesstimate my speed and how much gas is in the tank.

Well, when Michael, our first baby, was born, what was I thinking when I entrusted his father with the photography? I got him the simplest PHD—Push Here, Dummy—camera I could find. But did I think to load it? No. And neither did he. There he was, snapping away like Austin Powers, and I'm thinking, How cool! Someday I can show my son how he looked when he was a minute old!

Michael's birth was really easy. There was nothing unexpected. Except that empty camera. No, actually, I should have expected that, too.

Well, my sister is such a wise-ass. She lives in Phoenix and couldn't be there for the birth. She sent a really nice gift and also a beautifully framed picture of some kid graduating college. It's captioned "Ron's First Photograph of Baby Michael." I laughed and laughed.

For our other kids, I had a friend take the pictures.

Yes, I'm still married to Ron.

MEET THE PARENTS

Joan Hamburg, the host of WOR Radio's *Joan Hamburg Show*, a New York institution for several decades, decided she was going to give birth to a genius. Here's how she did it.

I have always been an avid researcher, so when I was pregnant, I devoured everything I could about childbirth. I clipped out articles on this oxygen machine that was being used by women in South Africa. According to stories in *Time* magazine and *The New York Times*, all the women in this control group were giving birth to genius babies. These infants were sitting up at five months old. They were talking and walking early, too. Also, the articles said that the women had very little labor pain. A genius and no pain, what could be better?

So I said to my obstetrician, "If you let me use this machine, I'll send away for it." He wrote a letter on his stationery and we waited for the machine to arrive. Unfortunately, it didn't get to me until the eighth month. The women in South Africa used it for at least six months before the birth, so I hoped my baby would catch up.

Well, the machine's really weird looking, but it claims to oxygenate the fetus. And because the baby's taking in this oxygen, he or she is supposed to be smarter than the average kid. You strap this gizmo around your waist, and by osmosis, your baby's sucking in this extra O_2.

So I wore it for the last month of my pregnancy. Then, when I went into labor on May 26, 1970, I wore the machine to the hospital. That's when my husband, Skip, started to lose it. He was saying, "Take the machine off her! It's crushing the baby. It's crushing her!" It was wild. He was really freaking out. With each contraction it felt as though my ribs were breaking. But once we got to the hospital, my son, John Liman, was born in an hour and it was a pretty painless birth. Remember, this was way before epidurals. He weighed 5 pounds.

There was this very large woman sharing the room with me and she was screaming bloody murder, so we gave her the machine. She wore it during the birth. We lost track of her, but I've always been curious to see what kind of kid she had and if he was a genius. Because, of course, our baby grew up to be brilliant. He's the kid who wrote the hit movies *Meet the Parents* and *Zoolander.* We always tell him the reason he's so clever is because he had all that extra oxygen as a baby. Maybe I should demand a percentage of his income.

UPSTAIRS/DOWNSTAIRS

Tim McGraw is one of the biggest-selling artists in the history of country music. Add his thirteen million albums and four million singles to the chart-toppers of his wife, Faith Hill, and the numbers become astronomical.

While Faith and Tim have much to be thankful for, they're proudest of Gracie Katherine, born May 5, 1997, and Maggie Elizabeth, born August 12, 1998. Here's Tim McGraw:

I admit I was nervous. I never thought about the actual delivery during Faith's pregnancies because we were always so happy, singing and talking to the baby and planning for its arrival. I would sing everything to Faith's stomach. Sometimes it would be my music, sometimes Elton John or Neil Diamond songs. I'd sing anything I thought they'd like during their time in the womb.

But suddenly in the delivery room, I started thinking about all the things that could go wrong. That was the most nerve-racking part for me—the way my mind just started playing out these worst-case scenarios. Faith ended up having C-sections with both girls.

Gracie was born three weeks early, so they had this preemie specialty team in the room. They took her over to the side and examined her. The whole time, Faith and I were holding our breaths. They handed her back to Faith and said, "She's perfect." In that moment we felt so much joy.

While we were in the room, I just talked to little Gracie. Since I sang and spoke to her before she was born, she knew my voice and her eyes followed me around the room. It was like she was saying, "I know you."

We didn't know we'd be having girls. It was a surprise. I have to say, it's great to be a daddy to girls. I'd love to have a boy someday, but it's hard to imagine how I'd be with a boy because girls are just so special. There's nothing like daddy's little girls.

With Gracie, we were typical new parents. We worried that if she was crying too much, something was wrong with her. Then, if she wasn't crying enough, we'd worry about that. During the first weeks, we didn't sleep. The biggest mistake we made was putting the nursery upstairs. We sleep downstairs, so for the first weeks we were constantly running up the stairs—nearly every five minutes. We checked her to make sure she was breathing and turned over the right way and not on her stomach. After a while we got smarter and moved everything—the crib, the changing table, the entire nursery—downstairs.

Faith and I want four or five kids—we want a house full of them. We'll probably end up with four or five girls. At least I'll be well dressed in my old age because they'll be trying to keep me in shape and fashionable, I'm sure.

Every night before Gracie and Maggie go to bed, we read to them. Lately, we sit with them and read a chapter or two of the Laura Ingalls Wilder *Little House on the Prairie* series. They look forward to this time. It's special for all of us, and they usually fall asleep listening to it.

We still sing to them all the time. They love music. The girls were singing before they were talking. Gracie can name any artist that comes on the radio. They like country music, but to be honest, they like the Beatles better.

WHO'S YOUR DADDY?

Craig Shoemaker is a comedian/actor/writer/impressionist ("My title has more slashes than a Wes Craven flick," he says). But he is best known as the Lovemaster, his signature character, also the name of the movie he wrote and starred in. Craig's one-man show, "Who's Your Daddy?," played to sold-out crowds in Los Angeles. An alternative to orthodox stand-up, Craig's show lays his soul bare, taking the audience on his emotional wild ride from "Lovemaster" to "Diapermaster." He shared his take on fatherhood with us.

*W*here do I begin? It's all so complex. My father left the family when I was one month old, so everything I'm about as a dad is being there for my son. I mean, I have some serious abandonment issues. If a waiter leaves my table, I ask him where he's going.

A few years ago, I got a second chance with a woman I'd once let slip away. So, the night she was packing to move back to Boston, I convinced her to stay in Los Angeles and give me another shot. She did, and a month later, she came out of the bathroom holding one of those little sticks that say, "You're pregnant!"

Well, coming from a broken home and having always yearned for a family of my own, my wish had come true. Trouble was, I had no road map. I had no idea how to go about being a dad. I had grown up in an all-female household. My first shave was with an Epilady.

So I set about trying to get ready. Having grown up with only women, I knew I was destined to have a girl. At one trip to the doctor, he did his sonogram thing and said it looked like a very healthy baby and did we want to know the sex.

"Oh, we already know. It's a girl."

"Really," the doctor said. "How do you know?"

"Well, from the way Carolyn's carrying, and we did the string test. It's definitely a girl."

"String test?"

"Yeah. You know . . . it's where you put a wedding ring on the end of a string and hold it over her belly and if it starts to swing counter-clockwise, it's a girl."

"Right," the doctor says.

Besides, when we discussed names for the baby, we both wanted "Emily," so that was further proof-positive kismet, we were having a girl.

We took the birthing class—it was the Bradley Method—at some woman's house, where we all practiced giving birth using a doll with a rope on it. But we didn't get to finish the class, because Carolyn went into labor a month early.

So, we're at the hospital and I'm telling her to breathe and push and she's grabbing me by the neck and choking me as she's screaming, "Epidural, epidural!" And I break loose and run into the hall screaming for Dr. Epidural.

Nothing is progressing according to my plans. Then nobody warned me what a new baby looks like, and when I saw the head I said, "Hey, you better put that thing back in there and let it bake a little longer." This is not what a baby is supposed to look like. It's bald with a point on its head. It's an alien.

But still I do my duty and coach, "Come on, Emily, come on, come on," and out comes a baby with balls—and I mean big balls—and I'm wondering what it's been doing in there for eight months with these tea-bag balls. But at the same time, I'm impressed. I'm thinking, "Okay, there's the wheels, now where's the cannon?" He's got these great big balls, but a little bitty nugget pee-pee. And I'm concerned. I say, "Doc, where's his penis?" And he says, "Well, it's a little small but . . ." And I say, "That's my wife's side of the family. They all have little dicks and pointy heads."

So all my plans and dreams happened but in their own time and way. I made sure that my newborn son had all the things I didn't have—both parents, nice house fully equipped, etc., but instead of coming home right away as I'd hoped, he was premature and had to spend his first few days in an incubator. I felt so powerless to help him. I wanted to swoop in like Super Dad, but all I could do was look at him through the glass. He couldn't swallow, and they couldn't find a vein in his little arm for the IV. This was not what I had in mind. I actually thought he wasn't going to make it. And then he rallied, and the next thing, we had him home.

Of course, the homecoming was not what I expected, either. He was up every minute, screaming. And let me tell you, everybody's got a solution for colic. I even tried putting him on top of the dryer. But somebody else said, "No, that'll give him shaken baby syndrome." And again I'd always figured when a baby cries, you just change a diaper or feed him or pick him up and comfort him and it stops. Nope. Another expectation blown to hell.

Just about when we got the colic situation under control, they throw a decision at me—circumcision. I figure, Okay, why not. My wife says, "Uh-uh."

Well, only in Hollywood. Our pediatrician, Dr. Fleiss (yes, that's Heidi Fleiss's dad, who is Jewish by the way), is very opposed to it. He says it originated as part of Abraham's covenant, which involved a two-part deal; sacrifice of your firstborn and circumcision, which was a way to mark slaves. Thank God, the firstborn clause was waived, but still, in Fleiss's opinion, circumcision is mutilation. And, he claimed that an uncircumcised penis was actually more hygienic.

But I'm still not convinced; I think a boy should look like his dad. And Carolyn asked if I'd ever seen my father's penis. Well, no, but then I went into the whole locker-room thing. So the days were quickly counting down until his circumcision.

I was doing *Hollywood Squares* and Whoopi hears about my dilemma and says she's researched it thoroughly and weighs in on the "don't cut" side of the argument.

Shortly after, I'm on *Howard Stern*, and he's very anti-circumcision. He starts dialing up doctors he knows and pals who had it done late in life and wished they could undo it. And I'm just freaked because all my life I never ever gave this thing a thought and now all these people are telling me *Don't do it!* Then I'm thinking, Jeez, my kid's life is gonna be in some way directed by Howard Stern!

Anyway, after all these messages, even though they were "Hollywood" messages, I figured I'd better listen. If I'd stayed in Philly, the kid would have been snipped. I guess he owes his "intactness" to Tinseltown.

My greatest fear is that my son emulates my life. I was a scrawny kid and I had colic, but I guess not having him circumcised begins to break the pattern. On the rare times that I was with my father, he was very standoffish—you know, "Hugging and kissing is for sissies; men shake hands with their father." Well, I'm throwing that bullshit right out the window. I kiss my baby boy to death. Sometimes I need a shave and I still kiss him like crazy. He must think, Here comes the human belt-sander. He's lucky I don't act on my impulses and take big bites out of him—he's that cute.

I waited a little longer to start a family, and I'm really glad I did. It's all just so precious to me. And I've taken on a fresh set of fears. I live in fear of anything happening to Justin. If he's playing in another room and I hear a crash, I jump out of my skin.

Since I'm on the road all the time, we have a nanny to help. Thank you, Joe Piscopo and Robin Williams, for wrecking the nanny thing for the rest of us. Thanks to those guys, only trolls need apply. When we were interviewing for nannies, anything over a six didn't even get the door opened. We have this nanny from South America. She won't speak Spanish to Justin, and I would love her to speak Spanish so he'll learn both languages. So instead Justin now speaks English like she does. "My name Yoosteen. I like to trow dee bowl."

One last thing about how kids change your life. Did you ever think you'd see the day when you'd actually volunteer to sniff someone's ass? I chase Justin around the house like some dog trying to sniff his ass to see if he made treasure in the Pampers. Crazy.

PAT BOONE'S "FOUR MISSES"

Besides being a show-business institution for decades, Pat Boone is one of those people about whom everyone says: "You just won't believe how nice this guy is." His career has spanned television, records and films. In 1997, he cut *In A Metal Mood*, putting the Pat Boone spin on hits from Alice Cooper to Led Zeppelin. And he even traded in white bucks for Doc Martens, black leather and a spiked dog collar.

Pat's proudest achievements are his four daughters. And in keeping with the ways of a dutiful and loving dad, he has a story for each one.

Shirley had gone into labor in the very early morning; it woke us both up and we headed for the hospital. Unlike other states at the time, Texas allowed fathers in the delivery room. So since Shirley's contractions were getting pretty close together, they gave her some kind of relaxant. She'd have a contraction, squeeze my hand till it subsided and then doze. Well, before too long, she starts to doze off, and since I'm having trouble keeping my eyes open, too, I just ask her to scoot over a little and I climb aboard the gurney with her. I just dozed between pains. When she'd get another contraction, I'd wake up and hang with her through it, and we'd nod off again. This went on for maybe a couple of hours until they became closer and closer and sleep was no longer an option. About that time, a nurse came in to check Shirley's dilation and said to me, "Okay, get off the table, Boone." I did, and then they went into action getting prepped for real.

I guess I was the very antithesis of the nervous dad. So, away they took my wife, and a little while later, we had this beautiful little 7-pound, 8-ounce girl—Cherry, we named her, for Cheryl-Lynn.

About a year later we were living in New York because I'd had a couple of hit records, and I had transferred to Columbia University in Manhattan. Before I graduated, we'd had Lindy, Debbie and Laurie.

Lindy came along on a Sunday. I remember that quite well because Shirley's water broke while we were in a church on the East Side of Manhattan. The hospital was downtown somewhere, and because Shirley's contractions were fairly far apart and we were both very hungry, we decided to stop for lunch on our way to the hospital. As we ate, we timed the contractions and then very calmly took a taxi to the hospital. That labor went on much longer—right through the night, and in the morning I went to class at Columbia and then came back just in time—but back then in New York, fathers weren't allowed in the delivery room.

Eleven months later, Debbie was born. The funny story there is, Debbie came a week or two early, and I was on the road playing some shows in Massachusetts. I'd asked a very close friend of mine, Don Henley (not of the Eagles), to stay with Shirley in case she went into labor. So when she did, Don took her to the hospital. They called ahead to our doctor and said they were on their way. The doctor was on the steps waiting for them and greeted Don (who looked nothing like me), "Hi, Pat. It's a pleasure to meet you. I watch your TV show all the time." Don had to explain that he wasn't me. A few hours later, Shirley had Debbie.

Laurie came right after Debbie, on the day of my live television show. I got to be with Shirley right up until the moment they took her into the delivery room. This was still before the days of Lamaze, I guess, and I would have loved to witness all four births, but the medical profession had other ideas back then. Laurie was a nice, easy delivery for Shirley, and that completed our family.

Each time I figured it would be a boy, and each of those girls was named Michael until birth. Shortly thereafter, having been thwarted four times in my efforts to have a son, I would kiddingly refer to my daughters as "my four misses." But they are, and will always be, my greatest hits.

15

Aftershocks

Some births are uneventful. Just wait a while.

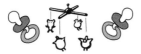

CLUELESS

Paul Takemoto resides in Kensington, Maryland, where he is a spokesperson for the FAA. Despite what you might think, he's actually a very smart guy.

Ben was our first and we didn't know what the hell we were doing. A lot of people just throw themselves into child books, but we didn't read a one of them. We went to some birthing classes but didn't really pay attention. So basically, it was like *boom!* little Ben was born. Actually, it was more like *boom!* baby Takemoto was born, because we hadn't even picked out a name yet. I guess we were in denial.

The middle name came to me in a moment of inspiration. After the baby was born, he was resting on my wife's stomach with his tongue lolling about. I looked up at the doctor, who was suturing Lisa, and he also had that tongue thing going. He had that deep-in-concentration look with his tongue sticking out the side of his mouth. It was like my baby and the doctor were mirroring each other. They really looked alike. That's how I came up with Benjamin's middle name. It's Thomas, after the doctor. I thought, Hey, someone's telling me something here.

After Ben was born, I told my wife I'd be in charge for a while.

She'd had a rough nine months, partially due to me. One day, about three weeks before the baby was due, I was outside pulling up weeds. I came in and the baby was kicking, so I rubbed my hands all over Lisa's stomach. I was following the baby's feet with my hands.

It turns out the weeds were actually poison ivy. My poor wife was covered with it from head to toe. She looked like a moray eel. It was August in Maryland and about ninety-five degrees out with ninety-five percent humidity. I'd come home from work and Lisa, who looked like she was having quintuplets, would have nothing on but a bra and panties. She'd be sitting on the couch, awash in calamine lotion, with the air-conditioning on full blast and a fan in front of her. She barely acknowledged my existence, since I was responsible for all of this—the baby and her itchy misery.

After Ben was born, I said it was my turn. I was a little crazy in the hospital. I asked the nurses hundreds of questions. For one thing, Ben's penis looked horrible after he was circumcised, especially with that torture device on the end of it.

So when does the clamp come off? Is it safe? Is that clamp going to be on him for the rest of his life? Will he have to take it off to urinate? I could hear his seductions: *Hey, baby, excuse me while I take my clamp off.*

After two days, I think all the nurses were glad to see me leave—they could rest a bit. When we got home, we didn't have anything except the crib. No diapers, formula or bottles. The only thing we had were those instant bottles from the hospital, and Ben had finished those off in a few hours. I had to run out to the store. I remember standing in an aisle just stacked with diapers and diapers. Huggies or Pampers? Premium or super? Regular or extra-absorbency? I never felt so overwhelmed.

Thankfully, I still had Jane. Jane was the nurse who had delivered Ben. Twelve years later, I can still see her face. She was an angel. Between four and five times a day for more than a week, I would frantically ring Jane for advice. After a few calls, I was on a first-name basis with all the labor-room nurses.

"Hi, it's Paul Takemoto. Is Jane there? . . . No. Oh, how about Helen or Carol?"

After a few more calls, I wouldn't even introduce myself. They'd just know.

"Hey, it's . . ."

"Oh, hi, Paul. I think Jane's assisting with a delivery, but let me see if she can take your call."

Most of my calls revolved around poop.

"Is it normal for Ben not to go for twelve and a half hours?"

"Yes, Paul."

"Yesterday it was like sesame seeds in a light soy sauce. Today it's like fried yams. Why is it different? Should we be concerned?"

"No, Paul. It's perfectly normal."

I wasn't a child father—I was thirty-one—but a little slow, I guess. I honestly believed that having a baby was akin to buying a refrigerator from Sears. If you had problems with the refrigerator, you'd phone the manager of the appliance department and he'd help you. Ben was still under warranty; Jane was the general manager of the baby department.

And then one day . . .

It had been over a week.

"Hey, it's me."

"Hello, Paul."

"Ben's umbilical cord just . . ."

"Paul, you know, our supervisor talked to us about your calls. We're really not supposed to be taking these calls from you. We're responsible for the delivery, but after that you're on your own. . . . I'm sorry."

I couldn't speak. I slowly hung up the phone. Lisa was watching me, waiting to hear Jane's sage counsel. "What'd she say?" Lisa begged.

I stared at her in disbelief. "She told me not to call anymore."

We just sat on the sofa, staring at each other and Ben, thinking, What are we gonna do now? What are we gonna do now?

We sat there paralyzed with fear. But soon Ben was crying and we couldn't think about it. We had diapers to change and formula to make. One day slipped into the next. A few times, I'd reach for the phone but stop myself. We were on our own. We were adults. We were *parents*. Then, one day, I didn't even think about calling. And soon I forgot the phone number entirely.

Ben's twelve now and I still have no idea what I'm doing. But maybe no one really does. We just fake it until we get really good at pretending. Anyway, Ben's great. He studies all the time and never gets in trouble. Now he gives me all sorts of advice. Too bad he couldn't have helped me out twelve years ago.

SHOW-AND-TELL

Betsy, a grammar-school teacher from Miami, remembers this Oscar-worthy birth tableau from one of her students.

I've been teaching now for about fifteen years. I have two kids myself, but the best birth story I know is the one I saw in my own second-grade classroom a few years back.

When I was a kid, I loved show-and-tell. So I always have a few sessions with my students. It helps them get over shyness and experience a little public speaking. And it gives me a break and some guaranteed entertainment.

Usually, show-and-tell is pretty tame. Kids bring in pet turtles, model airplanes, pictures of fish they catch, stuff like that. And I never, ever place any boundaries or limitations on them. If they want to lug it to school and talk about it, they're welcome.

Well, one day this little girl, Erica, a very bright, very out-going kid, takes her turn and waddles up to the front of the class with a pillow stuffed under her sweater. She holds up a snapshot of an infant.

"This is Luke, my baby brother, and I'm going to tell you about his birthday. First, Mommy and Daddy made him as a sym-

bol of their love, and then Daddy put a seed in my mother's stomach, and Luke grew in there. He ate for nine months through an
umbrella cord."

She's standing there with her hands on the pillow, and I'm trying not to laugh and wishing I had a video camera rolling. The
kids are watching her in amazement.

"Then, about two Saturdays ago, my mother starts going, 'Oh,
oh oh!'" Erica puts a hand behind her back and groans.

"She walked around the house for, like, an hour, 'Oh, oh, oh!'"
Now the kid's doing this hysterical duck-walk, holding her back
and groaning.

"My father called the middle wife. She delivers babies, but she
doesn't have a sign on the car like the Domino's man. They got
my mother to lie down in bed like this." Erica lies down with her
back against the wall.

"And then, pop! My mother had this bag of water she kept in
there in case he got thirsty, and it just blew up and spilled all over
the bed, like *pssshhheew!*"

The kid has her legs spread and with her little hands is miming
water flowing away. It was too much!

"Then the middle wife starts going *push, push* and *breathe,
breathe.* They start counting, but they never even got past ten.
Then, all of a sudden, out comes my brother. He was covered in
yucky stuff they said was from the play-center, so there must be a
lot of stuff inside there."

Then Erica stood up, took a big theatrical bow and returned to
her seat. I'm sure I applauded the loudest. Ever since then, if it's
show-and-tell day, I bring my camcorder—just in case another
Erica comes along.

IF YOU SO MUCH AS YAWN, I'LL SMITE THEE!

Elizabeth Michaels, a financial planner from the suburbs of New York City, had a surprise pregnancy that rocked her firstborn's world.

Artie and I had our first child, Gabrielle, when we were in our mid-twenties. By the time she was about two and a half, we decided we wanted another. So we tried. And tried. But it wasn't happening. And we were in agreement that if God didn't grace us with another baby, that was okay. We weren't going to move heaven and earth or go through any medical procedures to make it happen. We felt that children are a blessing, and we were grateful to be graced with little Gabby.

After a time, we just forgot about a sibling. Besides, we were too busy enjoying Gabby to think about much else. We run a small business from our home, so we had the luxury of watching Gabby grow minute-by-minute. And she had unlimited attention from Mommy and Daddy. Especially Daddy. You know what they say about fathers and daughters, and, boy, is it true. They were inseparable. Even when she was just a few weeks old, if he had to run an errand, he'd put her under his arm like a football, strap her into the car seat and away they'd go, laughing like drinking buddies. Artie could make her laugh like I never could. She would lose control to the point where the laughs turned to screams and shrieks. They were two maniacs.

Then, when she was about five, I became pregnant again. We were thrilled! We told Gabrielle she was going to have a sister or brother (we like surprises) that she could play with and take care of, and she was just as excited as we.

When little David was born, it was a snap. I don't think I was in labor for more than two hours—a very easy delivery. Artie was with me, but we didn't think Gabby was ready for the whole birth scene, so we stashed her with my sister for the day.

When we brought David home all bundled up, Gabby was crazy with excitement. "Let me hold it! Let *me* hold it!" I knelt down and put a sleeping David into Gabby's little arms, keeping mine beneath hers, just in case. Gabby got wide-eyed and silent. She put her face very close to David's and said, "He smells nice." Then she inhaled deeply and with all her might shouted, *"Hey!"* into his face. Needless to say, he was bawling instantly.

Artie and I didn't know what to make of that scene, so we just quieted the baby, gave him a bottle and put him in the bassinet. He was a great sleeper. He must have slept twenty-two hours a day the first few weeks. That is, after we kept him separated from Gabby. She was fascinated with him but also a little jealous of him.

If we let her, she would get up on tippy-toe and push a finger into his mouth, looking for teeth, I suppose. He'd be in his high chair, sucking a bottle, and she'd chew her food in his face. She'd pinch his bare feet. She'd hold his nostrils closed.

The complaints started. "You said I could play with him! He can't play . . ." How do you explain patience and time to a child who puts a card to Grandma in the mailbox and then asks if she got it before you get to the corner?

Artie and I had to be really careful to show Gabby her usual dose of attention. It was clear she was disappointed by the baby— we didn't want that turning to resentment.

After a while, I started playing on Gabby's maternal instincts, and she had them, big time. Some of it was maternal, but lots of it was her chance to be bossy, and let me tell you, she was a little dictator. For hours on end, I'd listen to her lecture her brother. "You need to finish your bottle. Help me pick up your toys. We're not watching *Barney*, we're watching *Sailor Moon*. Let's get your socks pulled up." God forbid he'd doze off in the middle of one of her tirades. "David Michaels, pay attention! You mustn't nap until I say so. If you do, I shall smite thee!"

I don't know where the hell she came up with the "smiting" stuff. Probably from those goofy Saturday-morning *Skeletor* cartoons or whatever. Seems like they're always smiting and avenging one another.

After a few months, Gabby calmed down and really started being helpful. We'd fold David's outfits or shop for new ones at Baby Gap. I remember when we bought him his first pair of shoes, she kept pressing the toes to be sure they fit right. She was really into whether he was ready for Pampers 3 or 4. And she seemed to have forgotten all about "smiting" him.

Now she's ten and he's five. She watches over him like a mother tiger. She's really protective of him, and that's great for us. But she's still a tyrant. Artie and I are really curious to see how David matures. He's either going to wind up a bachelor forever or some woman's slave.

AT LEAST HE DIDN'T SAY GLADYS BERTHA

Stan Taffel of Van Nuys, California, is an actor as well as a trainer and teacher for Gymboree, a play program for kids. Although he doesn't have his own children—yet— he had a big role in a friend's childbirth.

One of my favorite episodes of *The Dick Van Dyke Show* is where everyone is trying to name Rob and Laura's son, Ritchie. Everybody had definite plans—her side of the family, his side of the family, their friends. So they eventually settled on the middle name of Rosebud, which is a combination of a bunch of people's initials. It appeased everybody. I always thought, Wouldn't it be fun to name a kid?

Anyway, I was living in New York City when my friends Miguel and Jean were having a baby. Miguel's an actor and he was performing somewhere. So when Jean went into labor, she called me to meet her at the hospital.

It was the middle of the night and I was half asleep as I drove from the city to somewhere in New Jersey. I was so exhausted, but I wanted to be there for Jean. I didn't know what to do, but I tried to handle it the way Ricky Ricardo and Dick Van Dyke did. You know, real smooth. I even had cigars with me. I wasn't in the delivery room with Jean, but I was outside pacing the floor with all the other dads and relatives waiting for babies to be born.

As we waited, a nurse or two would come in. We'd all stand up in anticipation. Then the nurse would announce a name of a mom who'd given birth. Those who weren't there for that mom would all sit down again.

Hours and hours went by and no nurse came out to say that Jean had given birth. I ended up falling asleep on the couch. Hours later, a nurse eventually tapped me on the shoulder and said, "Miguel." Groggily I replied, "Yeah." After all, I was there for Miguel. The nurse goes, "It's a girl." I said, "Wow." Then they brought me to the nursery and I got to see her, which was amazing. The nurse goes, "She's beautiful. Do you have a name for her?" I just stared at the baby and out popped "Lindsey Rebecca."

Honestly, I was half-joking and half-asleep. I think I was just trying to put a combination together that sounded pretty and that I'd never heard before. If my brain was a roulette wheel spinning and each number had a name, I just stopped the roulette wheel on Lindsey and Rebecca.

I went in and checked on the mommy, who was exhausted but glowing. Soon Dad arrived and we hugged and hugged. I pulled out the cigars, but they'd gotten crushed when I fell asleep on them. Then I headed home and hopped into bed.

But just as I was drifting off to sleep, the phone rang. I picked it up and without even saying "Hello," Miguel goes, *"Lindsey Rebecca?"*

I'm completely baffled. "Huh?"

"You named my daughter Lindsey Rebecca?"

"What are you talking about? Oh, that? I just threw out a name. I was kidding around."

"Well, keep laughing, 'cause that's what they filled out on all the forms. So I guess that's what we're naming her," Miguel said.

They probably could have changed the moniker if they wanted to, but Lindsey Rebecca just stuck. I became her godfather and at the baptism, the priest goes, "What is her name?" In unison we said, "Lindsey Rebecca," in the same loud, sneering tone Miguel had used on the phone with me. I'm sure the priest was a little confused.

Even though everyone calls her Lindsey, I sometimes still say Lindsey Rebecca. She calls me Uncle Stan. One day I'll tell her the story of how she got her name.

PAIN IN CAPITAL LETTERS

Phyllis Diller is a pioneer in comedy. Preceded by many "comedic actresses," she was among the first women ever to take a stage alone and perform stand-up. The acclaim she met was immediate and lasting. While blazing this show-business trail, she raised five children.

Phyllis says there's nothing funny about childbirth. We're not so sure.

It was nothing but pain. Pain, pain, pain, like I never knew in my life. P-A-I-N in capital letters.

Let me tell you, there's nothing funny about giving birth. So of course you need drugs. Anyone who says otherwise is crazy. My advice is drugs. Take all the drugs you can. Oh, please, none of this natural childbirth stuff. My children were born before they invented Lamaze. There was pain then and there's pain now.

My labors were *loooooong*. Long and long. People say after the first child, it gets easier, but I think they say it to keep you reproducing. They were all painful and all hard. I had two boys and three girls. They were all difficult. I'm sure I made a lot of noise. I probably screamed. My husband was no help at all. He practically wanted sex on the way to the hospital, or at the very least the night before. I hated every minute of giving birth.

Okay, I shouldn't say that because once they came out they were so pretty and so cute. They were these really pretty babies and they all looked alike. The minute they came out, I loved them. I forgot all about the pain.

I had never really seen a baby and I didn't know how to do anything. The nurses had to teach me about bathing. I didn't know how to diaper—we had cloth diapers back then. For a while, I just threw away the shitty diapers. I'd take one look at it and say, "I can't handle that." Then I started running out of diapers, so I figured I'd have to suck it in and wash them. I even took a picture of my first diaper line. I washed them all and hung them to dry. I was so proud of that diaper line. It was tough, but I did it. I still have that picture somewhere.

When I was a girl, I loved playing mommy with my dolls. All I wanted out of life was to be a mother and wife. I wanted a houseful of children. I wanted to cook and clean and hear the noise of children all over the house. There's nothing better. Even today, I'm happiest puttering around the kitchen. Things are slowing down a little bit, but I can still putter.

My greatest joy in life is my family. My kids are all in their fifties and sixties, but they're still my babies. I have a great extended family with four grandsons. I got what I wanted and it was worth all the pain.

LIKE THE MAFIA, ONCE YOU'RE IN . . .

This is the authors' birthing-class story—too bizarre to be believed. But again, it's Los Angeles.

Irene was pregnant with our first, and we were as green as two parents could possibly be. Urged to attend birthing classes by the obstetrician, we signed up for the recommended course. And a course it was—into another dimension. Being native New Yorkers, we're still taken aback by the interplanetary zeitgeist of some Los Angelenos.

The instructress put the "Oh!" in blonde and was as grounded as champagne bubbles. Her oration included constant eye-rolls, head-tilts and tosses. If stumped by a question from the audience, she'd press a lacquered nail into her perfectly dimpled chin, cock her head and go, "Hmmmmm!"

For the first five minutes, we thought she was in character as a valley girl. I actually considered referring her to a talent-agent friend of mine. But when the act continued into the second hour, we realized we were watching reality—no, make that surreality.

Nobody told us that over the duration of six two-hour sessions, there would be maybe three minutes of useful information. That left eleven hours and fifty-seven minutes ranging from instructional videos with the production values of amateur porn to eye-twitching textbook tedium to weird "encounter-group-esque" confessions from the very odd assemblage of couples in the group.

After the first hour of Mitzi's instruction, she had everyone sit in a circle, just like on *Romper Room*. We were asked to introduce ourselves and tell if we were expecting our first child.

Irene and I said hello, that we were expecting our first and that we wanted to be surprised so had not asked the sex from the ultrasound people. As couple after couple took the floor, we became convinced we had somehow ingested hallucinogens.

"Hi! We're Jason and Marie. I run a medical-supply company, which has grown nicely over the last several quarters. I have a fleet of eight delivery vans and forty full-time employees. And we'll be expanding into Riverside County next quarter."

"What the hell was that?" I whispered to my wife. She dug an elbow into my spleen. My whisper had been more like a shout.

Next was an attractive couple. The woman did all the talking. She was a recent immigrant and her English wasn't too precise. She gave a full account of her career in the computer industry. After that, she went into a blow-by-blow description of the complications surrounding her first pregnancy, which went something like this:

"With first baby, I was at trade show with company in Las Vegas. Became constipated, had enema. Then contractions! I come back to L.A., they say no labor, but give me enema. Then two weeks later I at trade show, Chicago, my feet swell, I go to emergency hospital, get enema. Then home—just bad cold. Three weeks later baby born fine, but I never have so many enema!"

Who asked for all that? It got better. One guy thought he was a stand-up comic. "If she can't have sex for six weeks, is it okay for me to masturbate?" Two other guys told everyone that their first children were born out of wedlock. They had abandoned them and their mothers and were hoping to do better jobs this time around. "I want to be there emotionally," each said, sniffling.

It was bizarre. One squirrelly little guy—Lloyd—furiously scribbled every word that fell from Mitzi's pink-glossed lips. If he fell behind on his notes, he'd raise his E.T.-like arm and request clarification. I recall two of his exchanges perfectly, because I nearly had an aneurysm trying to suppress my laughter.

Mitzi was discussing the hemorrhoids many women develop late in their pregnancy. She suggested anyone suffering with those nasty grapes swab them with a product called Tucks. Lloyd's hand shot up.

"Yes?" Mitzi asked.

"Is that T-U-X or T-U-C-K-S?"

Mitzi bit her lower lip, rolled her eyes and giggled.

"Lloyd, it's T-U-C-K-S."

I turned to Irene and told her, "T-U-X are for formal hemorrhoids."

Another time, Mitzi was explaining how to breathe through contractions and pushing. As she demonstrated the technique, she counted aloud from one to ten. A few minutes later, she counted from ten to one. Lloyd's arm telescoped like a car antenna.

"Mitzi?"

"Yes, Lloyd?"

"Should we count from one to ten, or ten to one?"

But that wasn't the worst of it. On the night of the first class,

Irene and I had written our names, address and phone number on a class list. Unwittingly, we had enrolled in the Birthing Class Instant Friends Lifetime Membership Home Harassment Program.

Our baby was barely four weeks old when the phone rang one evening around 7 P.M. My wife took it.

"Irene! How are you? It's Roberta from birthing class. We're having our one-month reunion, so I want to give you the time and place. You've also been volunteered to bring either dessert or pasta salad, which will it be? By the way, are your nipples sore?"

Irene, always quick on her feet, told a beaut of a lie about having to go out of town that weekend. But after that the calls came in—with marching orders—for two-, three-, four-, and then a six-month gala reunion.

Roberta's requests became more and more strident, nearly crossing into demands. Who was this woman? She spoke with us like we were lifelong friends or recalcitrant relatives.

We had attended all twelve hours of nonsense. We witnessed no interaction among the couples. When had all this bonding taken place? It was puzzling. What were the shared experiences that forged these instant friendships? Viewing the public access–caliber videos? Listening to Mitzi describe how, while demonstrating various birth positions to another class, she had ripped a fart like a tuba blast?

Maybe it was those final ten minutes of each session, when the lights were lowered to backseat-at-the-drive-in levels, and the moms-to-be lay upon pillows while we daddies-to-be—coached by Mitzi in her transcendental, spirit-channeler's voice—practiced massaging them into a blissful, pain-free delivery trance, just as we would in the heat of parturition. Had there been more going on than Irene and I sussed under the fifteen-watt glow? Had there been some covert swinging we failed to notice?

After the six-month reunion phone message (we learned to screen all calls after 7 P.M.), we were commanded to pony up ten bucks to pay for our Birthing Class Reunion Newsletter and "Where is the photograph of your daughter?" For a short minute, I considered grabbing the phone and putting a stop to it, New

York style. But I banished the thought after realizing that this was just too entertaining, in a pervy, car-wreck sort of way. Why stop it? We were too curious to see how long it would continue.

Finally, after a full, 365-day solar revolution, Roberta stopped calling. But we still screen all calls after seven. And silently hope she'll return.

ACKNOWLEDGMENTS

The authors would like to thank Catherine and Raymond Zutell; Jeannine, David, Paul and Cate Schwing; Joan Zutell; Julie Jordan; Sheila Carmody; Stan Taffel; Annette DeBois; Ceil O'Hara; Bridget Moriconi; Elise Kingman; Bill McGee; Peter Scott; Ed and Maite Wilson; Dr. Pat Alaggia; Georg'ann Cattelona; Debbie Boucher; Joanne Wilkinson; Julie Keon; Monica Rizzo; Steve Buckingham; Michele Lincoln; Elizabeth White; Marty Ingels; Glen Lyden; Brian Quinn; Carol Sloat; Kurt Wahlner; Autumn Latimore; Bill Jaris; Jessie Schmidt; Nancy Iannos; Christin Conklin; Devin Owen; Cynthia House; Aretha Ivy-Bruner; Amy Jones; Jolene Van Mulm; Bruce McArthur; Kristin Arnold; Ron Stone; Michael Eames; Susan McGorrian; Vrena Margolies; Vickie Bane; Belinda Mercado; and Trinity Buenviaje.

ABOUT THE AUTHORS

*L*arry Bleidner is the coauthor of *The L&L Bean-counter's Catalog.* A former award-winning writer for ABC and Time Warner's magazine division, he is currently at work on a feature film for Universal. His wife, Irene Zutell, is a freelance writer and previously worked for *People* magazine's Los Angeles bureau. They live in Los Angeles, California.

Do you have a birthing story you'd like to share? E-mail the authors at izutell@aol.com.